Janet Jaffe, a pioneer in reproductive trauma, offers bereaved parents validation, compassion, and hope in her latest book. Drawing on real-life stories, research, and decades of clinical experience, she normalizes the complex emotions of loss and provides gentle guidance through the grieving process. With clarity and empathy, Jaffe honors the heartbreak of reproductive loss while illuminating a path toward healing, resilience, and growth.

—**RACHEL RABINOR, LCSW,** PSYCHOTHERAPIST AND AUTHOR OF *THE PREGNANCY AND BABY LOSS GUIDED JOURNAL*

In *Healing From the Trauma of Pregnancy Loss: Reclaiming Your Reproductive Story*, Dr. Jaffe's compassion, expertise, and commitment to grieving parents shines through from beginning to end. This book offers an empathic companion to parents who may feel alone and misunderstood in their grief and have no way of knowing how to mourn or how to make sense of their experience. This book is a much-needed guide for grieving parents on how to cope with the unique experience of pregnancy loss.

—**RAYNA D. MARKIN, PhD,** Associate Professor in Counseling, Villanova University, Villanova, PA, and licensed psychologist and founder, Therapy Center for Pregnancy Loss LLC

healing from the trauma of *pregnancy loss*

RECLAIMING YOUR REPRODUCTIVE STORY

healing from the trauma of *pregnancy loss*

JANET JAFFE PHD

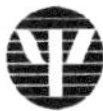 AMERICAN PSYCHOLOGICAL ASSOCIATION

Published by
American Psychological Association
750 First Street, NE
Washington, DC 20002
https://www.apa.org

Order Department
https://www.apa.org/pubs/books
order@apa.org

Typeset in Sabon by Circle Graphics, Inc., Reisterstown, MD

Printer: Gasch Printing, Odenton, MD
Cover Designer: Mark Karis

Library of Congress Cataloging-in-Publication Data

CIP data has been applied for.
9781433844416 (paperback)
9781433844423 (epub)
9781433849909 (pdf)

https://doi.org/10.1037/0000488-000

Printed in the United States of America

10 9 8 7 6 5 4 3 2 1

CONTENTS

healing from the trauma of *pregnancy loss*

INTRODUCTION

WHEN THE PATH TO PARENTHOOD IS THWARTED BY LOSS

If you are reading this book, you have suffered a loss that is heart wrenching and deeply painful, or perhaps someone very close to you has had this experience. For this, I am so sorry. Whether you are recovering from a miscarriage, a stillbirth, an ectopic pregnancy, the loss of a newborn, or a failed cycle using assisted reproductive technology, you have been through a trauma that is unlike any other. This is not only true if you have had a pregnancy demise, but it is also the case if you have experienced a failed adoption. This too is a pregnancy loss for the adoptive parents. It is also the case that medical circumstances may necessitate the termination of a pregnancy. For example, you may have had a medical condition that would negatively affect either you or the fetus if the pregnancy were to proceed. Or if you have had a multifetal reduction (e.g., a twin pregnancy reduced to a singleton pregnancy) for the health of the remaining fetus, you have had to make choices that are overwhelming and heartbreaking. Wanting a baby and then having to say goodbye to that child—or your hoped-for child, whatever the circumstance—is devastating. This book will help you and your loved ones navigate these losses and find a path forward.

In my work as a psychologist, I have accompanied individuals and couples—regardless of gender or sexual orientation—through this tragic time. I have witnessed clients in the depth of their despair, and I have helped them grieve, cope, and heal from pregnancy loss. I know how reproductive losses can shake the very foundation of people's lives. What we thought would be a given—the dream of having a baby and creating a family—vanishes into thin air. Not only do I know about this from the work I do, but I also know it because I too have gone through my own reproductive losses. In this volume, I hope to share with you my professional as well as personal knowledge of ways to work through this trauma.

As you dive into this book, you will understand why pregnancy loss is so traumatic. It impacts every aspect of our lives. If you have a partner, you may not be seeing eye to eye, with each of you coping and grieving in your own separate ways. Simple things like deciding what to have for dinner can suddenly become overwhelming. Making plans with family or friends may leave you filled with dread, as others often do not understand the extent of what you are experiencing. Indeed, they may try to be helpful and offer advice, but often their well-intentioned suggestions sadly miss the mark. You may shrink from checking social media, for fear that someone else will announce their pregnancy or the birth of their child. Without the possibility of moving to a deserted island, we must learn to cope with life continuing around us, even when our own life feels like it has stopped.

Although I cannot promise that this book will eliminate all the pain that you are feeling, I hope that it will help you feel supported and provide you with some pathways forward. This book is not meant to be a substitute for medical advice or therapy. Consulting with your medical practitioners about your situation and questions you may have is a must. Seeking the care of a mental health provider or a support group (see the Resources in this volume) is also recommended. This book, however, is meant to serve as a companion when you are searching for guidance—perhaps in the middle of the night, when you may feel isolated in your grief. It can help you find your way when you are feeling lost and alone. Some exercises are provided but certainly not required. This is a journey for you to take in your own time, in your own way. Perhaps this book will help you communicate with others around you so that they too can better understand this heartbreaking loss.

It is important for you to know this: No matter what you have experienced, you have been a parent throughout your pregnancy or adoption experience. The task ahead is to continue honoring yourself and your child in the best way you can.

A NOTE ABOUT LANGUAGE

Throughout this volume, I use the terms *men* and *women* for simplicity; however, it is understood that gender is on a continuum. Not all individuals who can bear children identify as female. Because of the physical demands of pregnancy on the female body, there is naturally attention to addressing women's psychological states; however, this volume will address men's emotional reactions as well, which are often overlooked. Additionally, while I may refer to *couples* and *partners*, many of you may not be in a committed relationship. Likewise, although I believe that the reproductive stories of members of the LGBTQ+ community as well as single parents by choice should be integrated in the heteronormative reproductive world, this volume will also attend to the special needs of these groups.

OVERVIEW OF THIS BOOK

The following is a chapter-by-chapter snapshot of what you will learn. Stories from many people who have experienced reproductive trauma and loss are provided in this volume. Please note that although the struggles are real, these cases are fictionalized to preserve confidentiality. In addition, you will find exercises throughout the book, which are meant to help you clarify your thoughts and feelings. As you will see, some of the exercises suggest you write things down; yet if this is not something you wish to do, just thinking about the suggestions works as well. It is the deliberate contemplation of the events surrounding your loss and what it means to you that enables you to heal and grow.

Chapter 1: When the Loss of a Pregnancy Becomes Real

Chapter 1 presents the concept of the reproductive story. Simply stated, the *reproductive story* is about all our hopes and dreams about having children. As will be discussed, everyone has a reproductive story, regardless of culture, race, religious orientation, or relationship status, including whether you are single, in a committed relationship, straight, or a member of the LGBTQ+ community. When the story goes awry—when the dreams of parenthood turn into nightmares—is the focus of this book. This chapter describes many reproductive losses that can occur. Although you are welcome to read through all the losses here, you may also want to focus on the issues salient to you. The nightmares people experience are not just about the physical demise of a pregnancy; they also include potential disruptions in relationships, as well as legal, ethical, and financial injustices. Indeed, as will be addressed, current restrictions in women's health care in the United States have only added to the trauma, making a bad situation even worse (Ranji et al., 2024).

Chapter 2: Your Reproductive Story: How It Began and the Chapter You Are in Now

Your story—how it began and how it developed over time—has many influences. Likewise, if you have a partner, they will have a story of their own that may not always align with yours. Chapter 2 encourages you to write down or tell your story as it was before the loss and then after. Once you can identify how significant your story is to your life, the depth of the blow when the story goes awry will begin to make sense.

Chapter 3: The Trauma of a Pregnancy Loss: What Happens When Dreams Are Shattered?

Pregnancy loss is a medical trauma as well as a psychological one. In Chapter 3, we talk about the assumptions you may have had about pregnancy—for example, that it is easy, and that everyone can do it. When these core beliefs are marred by loss, the solid foundations of your assumptions and all you anticipated you could count on are suddenly on shaky ground. Like rebuilding a house that has been damaged by an earthquake or flood, this chapter will guide you in restructuring your shattered assumptions and help you to build new ones.

Chapter 4: How Do You Grieve Your Baby?

In Chapter 4, we talk about grief in general as well as grief that occurs specifically in regard to reproductive losses. These are losses that can occur prior to pregnancy (e.g., in fertility struggles), losses during pregnancy, and postpartum issues. There is a misconception that the longer someone is pregnant, the greater the grief. It is, however, your emotional attachment to the pregnancy and the damage to your reproductive story that serves as a predictor of grief. We also explore the importance of rituals or ceremonies in the mourning process, and we discuss what you can do to memorialize your loss.

Additionally, grandparents-to-be, children who would become an older brother or sister, and other family members may agonize over the loss as well. They too have a story that is not moving forward in the way they had hoped. In fact, they may turn to you for guidance in their grief. This section discusses how to manage other people's grief as you try to deal with your own.

Chapter 5: We Are Not on the Same Page: When Couples Grieve Reproductive Losses Differently

If you have a partner, even though you share this loss, you may manage and cope with it in very different ways. The very person you usually turn to in times of distress—your partner—may not be emotionally available, bringing even more pain and isolation. This happens frequently in situations like these, and it doesn't necessarily mean that there is something inherently wrong with your relationship. In Chapter 5, through looking at other couples, we explore ways to better understand each other, increase your empathy for your partner, and learn more effective means of communication.

Chapter 6: I Feel Invisible: Coping in a Child-Centric World

There are so many emotional land mines to navigate when a pregnancy fails. Social interactions can feel overwhelming. If you have taken time off, returning to work can feel unsettling. Because people generally often do not know how to handle pregnancy loss, family members, friends, and coworkers can and do unintentionally say the wrong things. Chapter 6 offers practical advice as you deal with holidays, baby showers, weddings, birthday gatherings, and other social events. Your calendar, which may have served as a reminder for family birthdays or other celebratory events, may now be filled with sad reminders of due dates and the date of your loss. This chapter will help you manage your interactions with people who mean well but may actually cause you pain, and it will help you navigate those moments when you are reminded again and again of your loss.

Chapter 7: Trying Again: Hope Mixed With a Dose of Anxiety

Nearly everyone who has had a pregnancy loss lives with dread that it will happen again. How could you not be worried about that? Unfortunately, there is no way to pursue parenthood without taking the risk of trying again—whether that consists of trying to get pregnant again naturally, using medical intervention, or attempting to adopt. In Chapter 7, we discuss practical strategies to help you manage your anxiety and cope with this stressful time.

Chapter 8: From Reproductive Trauma to Growth: Healing and Change

The term *posttraumatic growth* (PTG; Tedeschi & Calhoun, 2004) refers to the potential for positive change following a major catastrophic event. This concept is as old as time: Out of adversity, growth will occur. As the words often attributed to German philosopher Friedrich Nietzsche (1888/2008) famously stated: "Out of life's school of war—what doesn't kill me, makes me stronger." Chapter 8 focuses on the positive ways you may change over time. The idea of time is of utmost importance here: Everyone needs time to heal. You will feel one way immediately after your loss and another after time passes. With that in mind, it will be helpful to do the exercises in this chapter now to note where your thoughts and feelings are currently, and then come back to the exercises at some point in the future to reassess changes in your attitude and perceptions of your loss. Doing so can help you see how you have changed and grown over time. PTG does not erase the loss—it is important to note that grief and growth can and do coexist.

Chapter 9: One Story Ends, Another Begins

At this point, we know how your reproductive story began and how it went off course. What you may not yet know is how your story will end—whether it will include children (or more children) or not. As we discuss in Chapter 9, finding different endings that bring fulfillment and meaning is the goal. No matter how your story ends, the loss has changed you in profound ways. It cannot be erased, but it can lead you in directions you otherwise would not have followed.

Epilogue: The End of the Story

All stories have a beginning, a middle, and an end. Right now, you are likely in the middle of your reproductive story, perhaps unsure how it will end. You may wonder if you will be stuck in this painful middle-of-the-story spot forever. Whether your reproductive story ends with having children or not, it is my hope that this book helps you move forward in your life.

CHAPTER 1

WHEN THE LOSS OF A PREGNANCY BECOMES REAL

We all have stories to tell. A story may reflect on something you did today, perhaps something to do with work or a conversation you had with a neighbor. Or you may tell a story about something that has happened in your past, such as a story about a colorful relative in the family, a happy memory, or a tale that leaves an ache in your heart. We tell our partner, family, and friends about the events that occur, and we listen as they too tell stories about themselves. Imagine that you are meeting someone for the first time. What story will you tell them about yourself? Perhaps you'll tell them where you are from or what you do. Narratives like these are so deeply ingrained in us that we tell them without effort as we disclose parts of the experiences we have had. While the stories we tell are often of things that have happened in the past, we may also share thoughts about the future—what we hope for and dream about. Research tells us that turning the events of our lives into stories is what makes our lives meaningful (Hydén, 2010).

Remember being asked as a kid: "What do you want to be when you grow up?" Think about what you thought back then; is it the same, or did it morph over time? For children, the dreams about becoming an adult and all the possibilities that the future holds may seem limitless. Kids may want to be an astronaut one day, a ballet dancer the next, or a doctor, an engineer, a superhero, a chef—you name it: The prospects are unbounded. For most of us, we hone in on our dreams, depending on our skills and the opportunities afforded to us. Ideas about what we want to be when we grow up change over time. The goals we set—whether they are related to career, creative endeavors, or relationships—and how we go about achieving them are what make up the stories of our life.

THE REPRODUCTIVE STORY

An important, significant, and universal chapter of our life story is that of parenthood. Reproduction is a part of everyone's life, regardless of race, religion, culture, gender, or sexual orientation. Even those who don't want children have a reproductive story. In essence, the *reproductive story* is the narrative of what we imagine it might be like to become a parent someday, or not (Jaffe, 2024; Jaffe & Diamond, 2011). We all wonder what it will be like to have children or what it will be like if we decide not to go down that path. That contemplation of the question "What is life going to be like?" is at the core of each person's reproductive story. The reproductive story begins in childhood; it morphs and evolves as we develop into adults. In Chapter 2, we'll see how the reproductive story develops and changes over time. For those of us who do want children, running into a roadblock along the way can be traumatic; it is a challenge like no other.

The reproductive story may include very conscious details: Maybe you thought about how many kids you wanted to have, or you imagined what gender they would be. Maybe you even picked out their names. You may have even chosen a career that would be family friendly—perhaps you wanted to be a teacher so that you could have the same schedule as your kids. The reproductive story includes all the hopes and dreams of what you imagine it will be like to have children. This story includes how we see ourselves as nurturing and loving, and it also includes the hope that our children's lives will be fulfilling and that their dreams will come true. Sometimes the narrative can be thought of as more like a picture book, with snapshots of your future showing you playing with your kids or passing holiday traditions down to the next generation.

Although the reproductive story may be vivid and conscious for some, the story may be murkier for others. That is, it may be more like an intangible and unconscious knowing that having a family of your own will happen someday. Maybe you weren't so sure you wanted kids. Lots of people feel ambivalent about it, perhaps worried they may not be up to the task. Some of us may feel we want to work on other goals—like finding a partner, pursuing an education, or establishing a career—before the idea of creating a family becomes a possibility. This too is part of the reproductive story; it comprises all the thoughts, ideas, and questions we have about it. As mentioned earlier, whether we want kids or not, the basic question we all share is this: "What is it going to be like?"

For heterosexual couples, the imagined story of pregnancy and childbirth may go something like this: "All we need to do is stop birth control, and voila! We're pregnant!" For single people or members of the LGBTQ+ community, getting pregnant is more complicated and may require using a donor, a surrogate, or other medical interventions. But no matter what, once someone becomes pregnant, the story usually continues with optimism: "Soon we'll have a happy, healthy baby in our arms!" The shock and trauma when the story does not unfold as we imagined is emotionally overwhelming and devastating for everyone.

Like many of us, you may have not even been aware your reproductive story existed—it is so deeply embedded in your core—until you experienced a pregnancy loss. Suddenly the dam breaks. Instead of what should have culminated with you holding and caring for a baby, you are now left with empty arms, empty cradles, and no lullabies to sing. When the reproductive story ends with loss, the trauma delivers an enormous blow to our sense of self. As we discuss this more throughout the book, you will realize this loss is a disruption that affects every aspect of life, from feelings about yourself to ruptures in your relationships, from feeling competent to feeling hopeless, from being able to count on tomorrow to feeling like all is lost. Feeling overcome with emotion, not knowing which end is up, is a normal reaction to this devastating trauma. You also need to remember that where you are now and what you are feeling now will change over time. You are currently in the middle of your story, and perhaps you have no idea how it will end. As you continue reading this book, my hope is that you will be able to rewrite and edit your story in ways you may not have thought possible. Doing so will allow you to heal.

HOW DID YOUR STORY GO AWRY?

This section describes some of the common pregnancy losses that can occur, as well as the loss when plans for an adoption are terminated. Whether you are cisgender heterosexual or a member of the LGBTQ+ community or you are single or in a relationship, you have a reproductive story that has not gone as hoped. Sadly, many people experience more than one of these losses, with reactions that can be searing and acute.

Making matters even worse are the recent restrictive laws on abortion in the United States resulting from the U.S. Supreme Court decision *Dobbs v. Jackson Women's Health Organization* (2022) and other legislation (Ranji et al., 2024), as well as the push to define personhood as beginning at conception. Women who are undergoing a miscarriage, for example, and the providers who are helping them, may feel they are under more scrutiny than in the past.

Women may be accused of seeking (or for clinicians, providing) an abortion, when in reality they are struggling with a nonviable pregnancy. Similarly, if personhood and all the rights granted therein begins at conception, then donating frozen embryos to science or letting them thaw could be considered murder.

These laws are affecting women's access to reproductive care (*Dobbs v. Jackson Women's Health Organization*, 2022). There have been reports of pregnant women whose pregnancy has been shown to be unviable having difficulty accessing care, depending on the state they live in (Nandi et al., 2024). Many must travel out of state to get treatment for a miscarriage. This travel may be financially restrictive or impossible for many, especially if they have child care issues or will need to miss work. In these cases, not only are women devastated by having to terminate a pregnancy, but they (and their providers) are also made to feel criminalized by it. For those already devastated by the loss, the limitations placed on women's health care make a bad situation even worse (Ranji et al., 2024).

Miscarriage

> I started to worry when after 5 months I still wasn't pregnant, but then it happened! My breasts got so tender; I knew that was a good sign. I started spotting a little when I was about 7 weeks along, but my doctor said not to be concerned, that it was very common. But then one morning I woke up and I didn't feel that tenderness in my breasts anymore and, of course, I started to worry again. I'll never forget that day. It was overcast and cold. I hobbled to the bathroom feeling crampy. The spotting was heavier; I knew I was having a miscarriage, and my mood matched the dismal weather outside.

Any loss prior to 20 weeks of gestation is considered a *miscarriage*. Miscarriage is one of the most common events of pregnancy loss, occurring in approximately 15% to 25% of known pregnancies (Genovese & McQueen, 2023). The rate may be even higher, because many miscarriages happen before people realize they are pregnant. You may have had a heavy menstrual cycle that came late; without a positive pregnancy test, there is no way to verify whether this was a miscarriage or not. The rate of miscarriage also increases with a woman's age. For a woman in her early 40s, it is estimated that about half of pregnancies end in a miscarriage; by age 45, this rate skyrockets to about 75% (Genovese & McQueen, 2023). Although miscarriage is statistically common, when it happens to you, the numbers don't matter. Your hoped-for baby has been lost.

The increase in miscarriages with age is likely due to a woman's egg quantity and quality, both of which diminish with age. Here are the facts: Unlike males, who can produce sperm throughout their lifespan, a woman is born with all the eggs she will ever have—that's about 1 to 2 million (American Society for Reproductive Medicine, 2012). By puberty, only about 300,000 eggs remain. This is a normal process called *atresia*, where the ovarian follicles, which are home to immature eggs, degenerate and die. As a woman ages and heads toward menopause, it is not only the quantity of viable eggs that decreases, but the quality as well. The older the egg, the greater the risk of genetic abnormalities, and this decline in quality is what affects pregnancy rates and miscarriage rates the most (American Society for Reproductive Medicine, 2012). When people speak about the *biological clock*, this is what they are referring to. The biological clock is in its prime when women are in their 20s; by the time a woman is in her mid-30s, the clock starts ticking more urgently and more loudly. This biological system made much more sense when life expectancy was only in a person's 40s; it is now approximately double that. Many women today are not ready to have children until they are older. I have had many patients who have been so upset when their doctors label them as having a geriatric pregnancy—that is, a woman having a baby when she is 35 or older. Although 35 does not seem very old, it is according to the biological clock.

To be fair, although men can produce sperm throughout their life, there is also deterioration in sperm quality as men age (American Society for Reproductive Medicine, 2012). However, this usually is not a problem before a man is in his 60s. The shift in fertility for men is nowhere near as dramatic as it is for women, with the precipitous drop in egg quantity and quality.

Women often blame themselves for causing a miscarriage, with age being but one factor in self-blame. They worry that they did something wrong. Yet most of the time, miscarriages occur because the fetus does not develop correctly. Often the miscarried fetus has an extra or missing chromosome, which has nothing to do with your actions or inactions (American College of Obstetricians and Gynecologists, 2022). I have heard women say that they carried heavy groceries, mowed the lawn, vacuumed the house, or drank a caffeinated soda—and they blamed the miscarriage on these things. You name it—the list of things women blame themselves for in causing a miscarriage goes on and on. Sometimes it can feel better to find a reason and blame yourself (even if your actions had nothing to do with the miscarriage), because then you can make sure you don't do that activity again. It is a way of gaining a sense of control. We know, however, that miscarriages are not caused by having sex, being upset, working, or exercising (if you are healthy). Believe it or not, I can assure you that miscarriages are not caused by stress (American College of Obstetricians and Gynecologists, 2022).

If you have experienced a miscarriage, it may have occurred naturally, meaning that it happened at home without medical intervention. These natural miscarriages can take around 2 weeks for all fetal material to pass out of your body. It is important for all fetal tissue to be expelled to prevent infection or ongoing bleeding. Your medical provider can monitor you to make sure there is no fetal tissue left in your uterus. Other times, women may take medication to assist the process; this eliminates the weeks of waiting and bleeding, and it shortens the timeline for a miscarriage because tissue can pass within a few hours. Combining medications like mifepristone and misoprostol is a nonsurgical method to help the body pass the pregnancy tissue. Mifepristone blocks progesterone, a hormone that is needed for an ongoing pregnancy, while misoprostol works by inducing uterine contractions to help your body pass the pregnancy tissue (MacNaughton et al., 2021). These medications, which are also used for abortions, have prompted controversy in the United States, with the potential of hampering miscarriage care. To date, the U.S. Supreme Court has voted to uphold access to these medications (*Food and Drug Administration v. Alliance for Hippocratic Medicine*, 2024), but the ongoing battles over reproductive care are far from over. The third method to treat miscarriage is through a surgical procedure known as *dilation and curettage* (D&C). A D&C is typically an outpatient procedure done in a hospital or clinic. After anesthesia, the cervix is widened (dilated) to allow a small instrument into the uterus to remove fetal tissue. A D&C may be necessary if you have had a natural miscarriage or used medication and not all fetal tissue has been expelled. All these options should be discussed with your health care provider to make the right decision for you.

Whatever situation you have experienced, the physical recuperation is usually quick. The emotional response, however, is a different story and can take quite some time to process. Don't be surprised by how a miscarriage is affecting you. You have lost a hoped-for baby. Your reproductive story has taken a dramatic turn. As we will talk about in subsequent chapters, you have experienced a trauma, and you are grieving. Unfortunately, many people around you may not recognize the significance of this loss. Because of that, you may feel even worse, as if you should not have feelings of sadness, anxiety, and depression after a miscarriage. These reactions, however, are normal and to be expected.

Because miscarriage is such a common medical phenomenon, providers sometimes gloss over it—telling you not to dwell on it, trying to reassure you, and implying that it is not a big deal. Unfortunately, this well-meaning advice can backfire. If you are having intense feelings after your miscarriage, you are not alone. When a clinician minimizes your experience, it can seem as if your feelings don't matter. You may even feel like you don't want to return to that provider, and that is okay. What's important to remember is your emotions are valid. The experience of a miscarriage and all the losses connected with it can be traumatic.

Stillbirth

> I was 8 months pregnant with my first baby and over the moon with excitement. She would be here with us so soon! We were on our way to pick out a stroller when I felt a sharp pain and then a gush of blood. We changed direction and went straight to the hospital. That car ride there . . . it was torturous . . . a 10-minute drive that felt like 5 hours. And then when we got there, they couldn't find a heartbeat; we were beyond despair. They induced me to go into labor. The silence that filled the room after her delivery was deafening. The nurses were wonderful. They encouraged us to hold our little girl, Abigail, and spend time with her. I wanted so much to hear her cry. I'll never get to hear Abigail, and that haunts me.

Whereas a miscarriage is classified as a loss prior to 20 weeks of gestation, a pregnancy loss is considered a *stillbirth* if it occurs after 20 weeks of gestation. A stillbirth occurs when a baby dies in the womb. As with miscarriage, many women blame themselves when a stillbirth occurs and wonder what they did wrong. Just as with miscarriage, the causes of stillbirth are generally not related to anything you have or haven't done. Sometimes they are caused by an infection, sometimes the baby has a birth defect, or sometimes they are caused by a complication in the pregnancy, such as high maternal blood pressure (preeclampsia). There are times when a stillbirth is caused by an umbilical cord accident, in which the blood supply to the baby is cut off; this can happen when the cord ruptures or is compressed.

According to data from the U.S. Centers for Disease Control and Prevention (2025), the rate of stillbirths for White women in the United States is 4.7 per 1,000 births. Shockingly, the rate of stillbirths for Black women is 10.3 per 1,000 births. The racial disparity seen in stillbirth rates extends to maternal mortality as well, with the rate of Black mothers dying while pregnant or shortly after birth more than double that of White women. Although there are no physiological reasons for these higher rates, they point to disparities in health care, with better access for White women than women of color (Eldeib, 2023).

Like a miscarriage, having a stillbirth is a traumatic experience that is complicated by the process of delivery. Reactions can include any one or a combination of feelings, including anxiety, depression, withdrawal, anger, confusion, or guilt. The heartbreak of having breast milk come in without a baby to feed intensifies these feelings. This is not the way your reproductive story was supposed to go. More discussion of these symptoms and how to cope with them and grieve will follow in subsequent chapters.

Ectopic Pregnancy

> I was overcome with joy when my pregnancy test came back positive. Three weeks later, I was overcome by pain—it felt like someone punched me hard in the gut. I had never felt anything

> quite like that before. It was such a nightmare. I was in an elevator on the way to work, and I just collapsed to the floor. Believe me, the last thing you want to do is be face down on an elevator floor! I couldn't get up. Luckily, a coworker was with me and called for help. It was terrifying. One moment you are on your way to work, the next you are in an ambulance on your way to the emergency room.

In a normal pregnancy, a fertilized egg makes its way through the fallopian tube, and it then attaches and grows inside the uterus or womb. An *ectopic pregnancy* occurs when a fertilized egg attaches outside of the uterus. The most common place for attachment in an ectopic pregnancy is in one of the fallopian tubes, which is often referred to as a *tubal pregnancy*.

Although a woman may have typical pregnancy symptoms such as nausea and tender breasts, an ectopic pregnancy cannot progress normally and it must be removed. A common question is whether it is possible to move the implanted embryo into the uterus; it is not. Ectopic pregnancies can be extremely painful, and they are life-threatening if the fallopian tube ruptures, resulting in hemorrhage.

An ectopic pregnancy, if caught early enough, can be treated with medication (American Society for Reproductive Medicine, 2023b). An injection of methotrexate stops the cells from growing. Methotrexate is one of the first medications used to treat rheumatoid arthritis; because this agent can be used to induce abortion, it may be more difficult for women to procure at this time. Use of methotrexate for an ectopic pregnancy, where a health care provider is prescribing it for a medically necessary procedure, may be questioned by antiabortion advocates because this medication is technically used to terminate a pregnancy. Aside from medication, the ectopic pregnancy can be removed laparoscopically, with hopes of saving the affected fallopian tube. If the tube has ruptured, it must be removed and may require emergency surgery (American Society for Reproductive Medicine, 2023b).

If you have had an ectopic pregnancy, the loss of one of your fallopian tubes may impact your fertility, depending on the health of the other tube. Not only are you grieving the loss of the pregnancy and the loss of your story, but you are also possibly grieving the loss of your health and fertility. Having an ectopic pregnancy does not mean you cannot have children, but you may be at higher risk of having it occur again. You may feel that your body has betrayed you, as the biological mechanisms of your body (i.e., having the embryo implant in the uterus) did not work as they should have. The anxiety of having another ectopic pregnancy can be intense. Before trying again, the body needs to heal. Healing from the emotional anguish may take even longer.

Termination for Medical Reasons

> My wife went in for a routine scan to make sure the baby was on track and growing. I was able to join her for this visit. I was so excited about seeing the baby for the first time, and I am so thankful that I was there. The sonographer was pressing on my wife's belly after slathering it with jelly. It didn't take a medical degree to see that something was wrong—the sonographer's face revealed everything. We didn't know what was wrong, only that this was no longer a routine visit. The sonographer excused herself to get the doctor. My wife started to cry; I grabbed her hand and didn't let go as we waited to hear the news.

The word heartbreaking does not describe the anguish parents go through when they are faced with the decision to terminate a pregnancy because of a medical concern for either the baby, the mother, or both. *Termination for medical reasons* (TFMR) can be morally and ethically agonizing. Because TFMR often happens in the second or third trimester, these terminations—although legal in most U.S. states—can lead to intense stigmatization for the individuals having them and for their providers. This issue has become even more critical since the overturn of *Roe v. Wade* with the *Dobbs* decision in 2022 (Hendrix et al., 2023).

A pregnancy may be progressing as expected when a routine test reveals a condition, such as trisomy 18, which could mean that the baby would either die in utero or hours after birth. If this were to occur, it is possible to have another healthy pregnancy following this loss. In other situations in which TFMR is necessary, this may mean that it is too risky for the woman to undertake another pregnancy. For example, the baby may be developing perfectly, but the mother's health may be at risk: This can happen if the mother has preeclampsia, a condition that comprises high blood pressure, protein in the urine, and impaired liver and kidney function. It is very painful to lose a healthy baby in order for the mother to survive, but failure to terminate can lead to the death of both the mother and the fetus.

If you are told not to attempt another pregnancy, there are other possibilities for creating a family, including using a surrogate or adopting. Although it can bring solace to know other avenues exist, your story is clearly not going as you had thought it would. As will be discussed in subsequent chapters, changing course and using a surrogate or deciding to adopt necessitates grieving your original reproductive story and rewriting it. The loss here is not just about the termination of the pregnancy, but it also demands modification of your story, which will no longer include a full-term pregnancy and childbirth. While surrogacy and adoption can be great alternatives, they are costly and not without risk as well. The point, though, is that any shift in your story needs to be grieved before moving on to other possibilities.

Multifetal Reduction

> We did not expect this! This was our third and final attempt at IVF [in vitro fertilization], so we transferred the three remaining embryos. After so many failed tries, we were shocked to find out they all took. Now we are pregnant with triplets, and we don't know what to do. We've been coping with infertility for so long, and now suddenly we are hyperfertile. We are so worried about the health and development of these babies, never mind my ability to carry them or care for them after birth. We know there are so many risks involved. Our doctors talked to us about the chances of delivering early and the multiple risks that can plague premature babies for their entire lives. We don't know how to manage all this.

People in this situation are faced with complex moral and ethical decisions regarding *multifetal reduction*. Is it morally permissible in a multifetal pregnancy to terminate a viable fetus for social or financial reasons? What if it is necessary for medical reasons? Weighing the risks and benefits in the decision to either reduce the pregnancy or maintain it presents individuals or couples with overwhelming and profound choices. Added to that are the potential legal ramifications, with abortion laws differing from state to state in the United States (Brendel & Kennedy, 2023). Prior to the reversal of *Roe v. Wade* with the *Dobbs* decision in 2022, selective reductions were permissible under law. Current statutes, however, may restrict or prohibit selective reductions, complicating an already difficult decision (Brendel & Kennedy, 2023).

On one hand, a pregnancy reduction will cause the loss of one or more of the fetuses, and it may even cause the loss of the entire pregnancy. On the other hand, there are risks in not reducing. Multiple pregnancies often end with premature births, which can have dire and lifelong health consequences for the children. A reduction may increase the chances that the remaining fetus or fetuses will have better odds of survival and health. A multifetal reduction may ensure the health of the mother as well, as carrying multiples is riskier than carrying a singleton.

Multifetal reduction is a pregnancy loss unlike the others previously discussed in this chapter. This loss requires a conscious weighing of plusses and minuses; in other types of pregnancy losses, there may be no choices available. You may be weighing moral, ethical, and religious factors, along with practical economic concerns. If you have opted to do a reduction, it may be agonizing to decide which fetus to eliminate. Sometimes this becomes obvious, as one fetus may not be developing as much as the others. It is also possible to test the fetuses before reduction to see which ones are healthy and which may not be.

For some, the decision to undergo a multifetal reduction comes more easily. They know what will be right for their family. For others, however, this decision is agonizing. Sometimes it can be helpful to create a spreadsheet of the pros and cons of the situation; it can help to take the emotional triggers out of the equation and analyze the facts. Regardless of your decision, however, this loss must be grieved as well.

A similar situation is when there is a natural demise in a multiple pregnancy, with a surviving child. In this case, a decision about pregnancy reduction is not necessary, although it remains emotionally complex. For example, in a twin pregnancy, one fetus may die. If the death occurs early on, it usually does not have consequences for the remaining twin. However, if the death of a twin occurs in the second or third trimester, there may be medical complications for the surviving twin as well as the mother. Examples may include preterm labor, preeclampsia, and growth restriction for the remaining baby. Sometimes the surviving baby may die as well. The emotional toll this can take on the pregnant woman is enormous when both grieving a loss and hoping for a continued pregnancy with a positive outcome at the same time. Focusing on one fetus and not the other can feel wrong, as if somehow you are not caring for both children equally. Aside from the medical trauma, the psychological trauma, including anxiety, guilt, and a sense of helplessness and shame, needs to be addressed.

Failed Assisted Reproductive Technology

> This was our first time doing IVF. We were excited but anxious at the same time. What an arduous process! Our nerves were rattled: What if we did the shots wrong? What was it going to feel like to retrieve the eggs? We made it through all that and nine eggs fertilized!! But after testing the embryos, only two came back as normal. We transferred one with high hopes—our doc was very optimistic. But no luck. Yes, we have one more, but right now it feels as if everything we had hoped for is over. The thought of having to do another cycle of IVF is devastating—never mind the cost. It feels like we are back at square one.

Whether you are in a heterosexual relationship or a member of the LGBTQ+ community, you may need to seek assistance from a reproductive specialist to build your family, such as through IVF, a donor, or a surrogate. When any of these assisted reproductive technology interventions fail, people describe their experience as a loss. Even without a positive pregnancy test, the sense of loss is the same. One of my patients described her experience of having cells dividing in a petri dish as feeling "a little bit pregnant." Research has shown that the grief after a failed IVF cycle mirrors the feelings that women have after a pregnancy loss (Greenfeld et al., 1988). Here again, the reproductive story, with all the fantasies of a life with children, has been affected.

Because these kinds of losses may not entail any visible sign of pregnancy or a positive pregnancy test, they may go unrecognized.

The only people aware of the loss may be the woman, her partner (if she has one), and her doctor. Although it may be hidden in the shadows, the emotional and psychological distress is not diminished. In fact, because it may not be addressed openly, the shame, isolation, and self-blame may be even more intense. As you read on, it will become clear why these invisible losses are so distressing, and we will discuss how to cope with them and ways to grieve.

Surrogacy and Loss

> I decided to become a surrogate after my brother, who is gay, talked about how much he wanted to have kids. He and his partner would be such great parents! I knew I couldn't be a surrogate for them, but I could do it for another couple. Pregnancy and childbirth were relatively easy for me—both my children, now 3 and 5, are such a joy. I realized I could provide this gift for a gay couple or for a straight couple who couldn't have kids on their own. I didn't consider there would be any problems, as my own pregnancies went so well.

Surrogates—women who carry a pregnancy for others who are, for whatever reason, not able to carry a pregnancy themselves—are not immune to pregnancy loss. If a surrogate experiences a miscarriage or other neonatal loss, her grief includes not only her own sense of failure and sadness but also the weight of letting the parents-to-be down. The would-be parents are also grieving this loss—their hopes have been dashed. A surrogacy loss can compound the grief of would-be parents, especially if they had previous unsuccessful attempts at creating a family.

Because surrogacy arrangements require legal as well as medical involvement, the agreement can feel very contractual. The human element—the feelings that are involved between the surrogate and the intended parents—may get overlooked. It is important to remember that the surrogate and her family as well as the intended parents have suffered a significant loss that needs to be grieved.

Cancer and Reproductive Loss

> We were excited about starting a family. My wife went to see her gynecologist for a checkup, just to make sure all systems were go, but a diagnosis of breast cancer stopped us in our tracks. Obviously, moving forward with a pregnancy at this time was out of the question.

Most people do not anticipate that their reproductive story could be derailed by a life-threatening illness such as cancer. Many cancer treatments, such as chemotherapy or radiation, can cause infertility. While individuals are dealing with fears associated with their diagnosis, they also may need to make rapid decisions about preserving their fertility. For men with cancer, freezing sperm (collected by masturbation) before cancer treatment is recommended (Practice Committee of the American Society for Reproductive Medicine, 2019). For women, preserving their fertility is much more complicated. To freeze her gametes, a woman must undergo an IVF procedure, which may not be covered by health insurance and may delay the start of cancer treatment. Depending on the diagnosis, delaying chemotherapy or radiation may be contraindicated. Fertility preservation is a key survivorship issue for people of all genders (Angarita et al., 2016). The double blow of receiving a life-threatening diagnosis and the potential loss of fertility can be overwhelming.

Adoption Failure

> After several years of fertility treatment, we finally decided to adopt. The process was not easy. The adoption agency helped us prepare a brochure about ourselves—it felt so strange to

> have to market ourselves as suitable to become someone's parent! But we followed the advice of the adoption agency—took happy pictures of ourselves with our dog—and featured more pictures of our vacation hiking in the mountains. Would this be enough to convince someone that we are good people who could be trusted with their baby?
>
> When the call came that a birth mother had chosen us, we felt like we had won the lottery! Over the weeks of getting to know the birth mother, we were excited but also a little nervous. We recognized what a challenge this was for her, what a leap of faith that she was doing the best for her child. When she gave birth, we were in the waiting room. She called us in, and as soon as we saw her holding the baby, our hearts sank. We just knew she had changed her mind. All of us were in tears. She said how sorry she was, but she just couldn't let her little girl go. What a mix of emotions. We understood her pain and her decision, but we were devastated. Once again, our arms were empty as we longed to hold our baby.

The chance that birth parents—usually the birth mother—will change their mind is a risk that adoptive parents take. The grief and emotions that you as an adoptive parent feel are akin to that of other pregnancy losses. Like many people who have chosen to adopt, you may have struggled for years with failed fertility treatments, only to have your hopes dashed once again. In addition, you may have many complicated feelings about the birth parents—perhaps anger mixed with empathy. You may feel very alone when an adoption you were counting on doesn't go through. This is a loss that is rarely discussed but needs to be grieved just like other pregnancy losses.

Abortion

We now arrive at the controversial subject of abortion. The discussion here is not about whether abortion is right or wrong; rather, we highlight the fact that this too is a pregnancy loss. So far, we have addressed people wanting a child and not being successful at it. Those reproductive stories have clearly not gone as hoped for. It is also true that becoming pregnant under circumstances when it is unwanted is another way a reproductive story has gone awry.

Someone who has chosen to have an abortion may think that they are not allowed to grieve. The truth is that even when the decision may be clear and may be accompanied by relief, many other emotions can arise. Guilt may be one of them. Sometimes people feel guilty that they have found themselves in this situation at all. Perhaps it was just not the right time to start or expand a family, perhaps it was a mistake, or perhaps the pregnancy was due to incest or rape. Women may also feel a sense of shame that they find themselves in a circumstance that creates internal distress and chaos.

It would be simplest if, in all situations in life, we could respond with one set of clear-cut emotions. The beauty of human psychology, however, is that we can and do feel many emotions at the same time. How often have you felt angry at someone you love? The same is true with feelings about abortion. It is important to stress that to process this experience, feelings should not be stuffed away. As with other life crises, finding support and understanding and giving all the emotions voice will help lead to resolution.

REACTIONS TO PREGNANCY LOSS

All the losses described here have a common thread: The reproductive story appeared one way prior to your loss and another way after. The loss of the reproductive story can be likened to a rug being yanked out from under you. That is, everything you counted on (sometimes without even realizing it) is suddenly flying around and hasn't landed back in place. The things flying through the air are all your emotions, all your hopes and plans, and indeed what you imagine your future will be like. You may even wonder if things will ever get back to normal.

The ripple effect of pregnancy loss is huge. It acts like a stone being thrown into a lake, with waves of concentric circles billowing out. The central circle signifies the impact of the loss on you and your sense of self. It embodies feelings of anxiety, depression, and negative self-worth. The subsequent circles, as illustrated in Figure 1.1, affect your intimate relationships, family ties, and relationships with friends and coworkers and, finally, spread out to the child-centric world at large. Everything and everyone is touched by this trauma. Such is the force of a pregnancy loss and the loss of your reproductive story.

One of the many myths about pregnancy is that anyone who wants to can get pregnant—it is a natural part of human biology, after

FIGURE 1.1. Ripple Effect of Pregnancy Loss

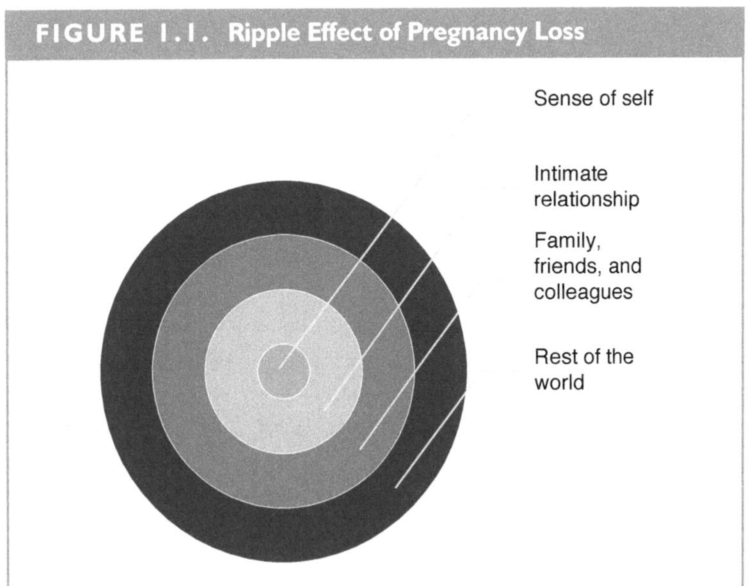

all. This is a common notion: It is easy, and everyone can do it. Ask anyone who works in reproductive medicine, however, and they'll tell you that even if you are young and healthy, you never can predict the outcome of a pregnancy—if the woman is able to conceive at all. It truly is a miracle when all systems line up to produce a flourishing newborn. Even if the odds are in your favor that you will have a positive outcome, it is something we should never take for granted.

Another common myth is that the longer you have been pregnant, the greater the emotional distress. This is also not true. The previous section described different losses that can occur and the physical and emotional fallout from them, but what is common to them all is that reactions are not predicated on gestational length. What does determine grief is the intensity of the attachment that people have with their unborn fetus or baby who has died. A woman who has had a miscarriage at 10 weeks, for example, may experience similar emotions to a woman who has had a loss in the third trimester. The bond that develops may be just as intense. In both cases, her baby has died. All the hopes and dreams she had for this child have suddenly vanished.

Think back to your reproductive story. This is where we can trace the beginnings of attachment. The bond you feel may intensify as a pregnancy becomes more real, but attachment can take place even without a pregnancy. As discussed earlier, IVF procedures that fail can be experienced as a death and need to be grieved. Research suggests that grief after a failed IVF cycle can be just like reactions after a pregnancy loss, with attachment to the pregnancy being the predictor of feelings of loss (Greenfeld et al., 1988).

Aside from attachment, other factors affect grief. One factor is whether this was a desired and planned-for pregnancy. A pregnant teenager who has ambivalent feelings about becoming a mother may feel very different about a miscarriage compared to a 35-year-old woman who has been eagerly anticipating parenthood. The teen may feel relief; perhaps she had thought about having children someday, but not now. The older woman is likely to be devastated; her hopes for a pregnancy and parenthood are on a very different timeline than the teenager. It is important to remember that both the teen and the older woman have reproductive stories that have gone awry.

It is heartbreaking to experience a perinatal loss (i.e., a loss before, during, or after pregnancy), and sadly, sometimes people experience more than one. If you have struggled with infertility and then have a miscarriage, it may feel that you are doomed and will never be able to have a child. While a pregnancy loss does not guarantee that you won't have another one, it also does not mean that the next pregnancy won't go perfectly well. In my many years of working with women and couples, I have witnessed the anxiety and trepidation of trying again. I don't think it is possible not to worry that a subsequent pregnancy won't be the same as the previous one. In my own experience, after several miscarriages, I was on guard throughout my pregnancy that was finally successful. This is normal and to be expected.

Your age can also predict the intensity of anxiety and grief. Women older than age 35, whose biological clock is ticking, are likely to have a stronger emotional reaction because they may feel that time is running out. There may also be a difference in your reaction if you have other living children. Other children won't protect you from feeling grief; but if you don't yet have children, you may feel more desperate and apprehensive that it will not happen. Perhaps there is added pressure due to other family dynamics. Some know they are the last hope of providing grandchildren. Would-be grandparents too have reproductive stories that extend to their adult children's reproductive lives. They may be grieving their own story about having grandchildren while grieving for you at the same time. After all, you are their baby, and they don't want to see you suffer.

SUMMARY

This chapter has introduced you to the concept of the reproductive story. It has touched on some of the various pregnancy losses that can occur. If you have found your own or a loved one's experiences in these pages, please keep reading, as you will learn how to mourn these losses, how to cope, and how to rewrite your story. In the next chapter, we'll discuss how your story began and how it developed over time. Once you identify how significant your reproductive story is to your life, the depth of the blow when the story goes awry will make sense.

CHAPTER 2

YOUR REPRODUCTIVE STORY: HOW IT BEGAN AND THE CHAPTER YOU ARE IN NOW

In this chapter, we will talk more specifically about the beginnings of your reproductive story and how it evolved over time. Recognizing that the reproductive story is so deeply ingrained in your identity gives insight into why these losses are so traumatic. Exercises are offered in this chapter: You can do them by writing down your thoughts and feelings, you can talk about them, or you can even just use them to prompt your thinking. Research suggests (as we will focus on in Chapter 8) that the more you deliberately reflect on the trauma, the more you will heal and grow (Tedeschi & Calhoun, 2004).

THE BEGINNINGS OF YOUR STORY

Picture a preschool: There will surely be lots of activities or play areas for children to choose from. There may be areas for kids to build things, stations for artwork to be created, and spaces with puzzles and books to explore. There may also be dress-up clothes to don, make-believe kitchens with pretend food, and maybe even cars for toddlers to sit in and drive. Can you think back to your own childhood? What were some of your favorite activities? I can remember a toy car, with a steering wheel, turn signals, and a horn, that I loved to drive. I also remember a very special red telephone, which I used to make official calls from my pretend office, and a Betsy Wetsy doll that I adored (if you are too young to remember Betsy Wetsy, she drank water from a toy bottle, cried tears, and, of course, needed her diaper changed). I recently came across a YouTube video of an old commercial for Betsy Wetsy (https://youtu.be/Kx4_1cL4M2s?si=dtcEhaKSYlYXe2vi). In the video, a little girl is taking care of her doll while the announcer says, "Ask your mommy for a Betsy Wetsy doll, and then you can be a mommy too." Without realizing it at the time, the foundations for my reproductive story and my fantasies about becoming an adult were being formed.

Make-believe play is a huge part of a child's life; it often centers on pretending to be an adult or engaging in adult activities. The toys that I played with are great illustrations of this: I pretended to drive, go to work, and be a parent. Children's play is the very beginning of the reproductive story. Play is a universal phenomenon, occurring across cultures, genders, religions, and races and ethnicities. Through play, children try on not only oversized shoes and clothing but also their imagined self as an adult and as a parent. As discussed in Chapter 1, the possibilities of what children believe they can do and what they might become may seem infinite. Indeed, the answer to the question "What do you want to be when you grow up?" may change from day to day. The constant throughout children's lives is the goal of growing up; incorporated into this goal is the idea of becoming parents themselves. In psychology, we call this the beginnings of children's *parental identity*, that part of oneself that envisions the role of becoming a parent. This parental identity is so central to our core self that we often don't recognize its importance until much later, such as when the path to parenthood is disrupted.

Because of conventional gender norms, it is often assumed that only little girls have reproductive stories that begin in childhood. It is easy to observe the beginnings of parental identity when girls play with dolls. Baby dolls are fed, dressed, bathed, and taken for walks in a stroller; they also may be scolded and told "no" for doing something wrong. This play often runs parallel to children's own experience of being a child. Children mimic what they observe and what they experience. Sometimes, children work through an emotional or troubling event during play. For example, let's say that a young girl fell while climbing a jungle gym and broke her arm. Her play may then incorporate rushing to the hospital, pretending to be the kind doctor who took care of her, and making sure her stuffed animal got a special treat when it came home.

Contrary to popular belief, reproductive stories are not just for little girls. This is a stereotype that, when looked at more closely, we know is not true. First, not all little girls like to play with dolls. Girls may be much more interested in rough-and-tumble activities but display nurturing behavior in other ways—maybe by helping another child put on their shoes, taking care of a pet, or getting a friend something to eat. The reproductive story does not always present as play being a mommy. Second, little boys have reproductive stories as well. For example, boys may play with dolls too or they may create a family of trucks or dinosaurs, displaying caring actions that mirror activities of their home life. For example, one little boy had a favorite toy rabbit that he kissed and tucked into bed each night; he could be found reading to his bunny before he knew how to read. Another boy had a tool chest with which he fixed things, as he identified with his fix-it dad. Other imaginative play, such as wielding a sword to save a castle from dragons or pretending to be a superhero and save the world from evil villains, can also be thought of as protecting and nurturing. This too is part of children's reproductive story.

Mental health professionals who work with children encourage play as a way to communicate without the need for verbal language. I once worked with a 6-year-old girl who gathered all the toys in my office into a small box. She said she needed everyone to be together. This was her attempt to work out feelings of loss over her parent's divorce and the disruption in her family. "Let's get another box and put it right next to this one," I suggested. "Then we can move some toys into that one so they're not so smushed up against each other. They need some room to move!" With great thought, she picked out the ones she wanted to move. She kept moving one of the toys, a monkey, back and forth from one box to the other. She then burst into giggles—so different from her somber, scared demeanor when she first came in—knowing that the monkey would be welcome in both boxes. "Everybody loves the monkey!" I declared, trying to reassure her that she would be loved in both her mother and father's new homes. Through play, she was able to step toward acceptance of the family's dissolution to a new family structure.

Children's play for both boys and girls is a cross-cultural phenomenon. Research on play has examined Western and non-Western societies alike and acknowledges that a major role of children's play is to assimilate their culture by imitating adult role models (Gosso & Carvalho, 2013). By pretending, children can integrate and incorporate the world around them. Regardless of country of origin, socioeconomic status, race, religion, or ethnicity, kids reflect on adults and play at pretending to be adults. It is this type of play, no matter a child's gender or their sexual orientation later in life, that sets the stage for this question: "What will it be like when I grow up?"

Exercise 2.1 encourages you to revisit your memories of childhood. Doing so will help you think about the beginnings of your reproductive story.

EXERCISE 2.1. A Trip Down Memory Lane

As you have been reading through the earlier descriptions of how reproductive stories begin, you have undoubtedly been thinking of your own childhood. Memories may come flooding back. What were your favorite

EXERCISE 2.1. A Trip Down Memory Lane (*Continued*)

toys? What were your favorite activities? Did you like to help around the house by vacuuming or gardening with toy replicas of the real thing? Take a moment and think about the beginnings of your story. If you are so inclined, it can be helpful to write these remembrances down and share them with your spouse, your partner, a trusted family member, or a friend.

Your parents or siblings may have recollections of your childhood that can add details to your story. Talking about your memories of childhood with them will likely trigger their memories not only about your childhood but their own as well. You may want to ask them about their reproductive story. What were your mother's favorite toys, for instance? Having insight into what those close to you imagined can make you feel even closer to them. Some of these memories may make it clear what your dreams have been, and perhaps they are the exact things you imagined your hoped-for children will experience someday.

Of course, not all memories of childhood are positive. The reproductive story, however, is based on what you hope for when you become a parent. The story may include thoughts and feelings about what you don't want for your imagined child. Perhaps part of your story includes things like this: "I will never hit my child," "I won't yell at them if they've done something wrong," or "I won't force them to finish everything on their plate." Your story is aspirational, wanting what's best for your child-to-be.

These snapshots of our early childhood help lay the groundwork for the rest of our lives. In reflecting on early memories, can you see the connection to where you are now as an adult? We will talk next about how early play morphs and develops as we get older. But for now, wind back the clock and indulge in your memories.

YOUR REPRODUCTIVE STORY DEVELOPS OVER TIME

The toys of childhood are replaced with other interests as we get older. Indeed, the events of adolescence and early adulthood continue to shape our reproductive stories. As our bodies mature and ready us for parenthood, so do our psyches. Just as in early childhood play, we try on different adult personas. Adolescence is a great example of this. It is a time of experimentation, attempting to understand just who we are and what we may become. The psychological term for these developmental phases is *separation/individuation*. It has been theorized that there are three separation/individuation phases in our lives: the first occurring in early childhood (Mahler et al., 1975), the second in adolescence (Blos, 1967), and the third in the process of becoming parents (Colarusso, 1990). Each phase is highlighted by extensive physical, psychological, and social and emotional growth. These phases are often referred to as *crises*, meaning from a relatively stable growth period there is a sudden leap forward. As will be discussed, when an actual crisis occurs within a separation/individuation phase (e.g., a pregnancy loss), that leap forward can feel as if you have crashed into a brick wall, with deep injuries to your sense of self.

What are some of the factors that can influence our development from childhood through adolescence and then into adulthood? How do these circumstances shape our feelings about parenthood? So many things can play a part. As we've discussed, one critical aspect is our relationship with our parents and caregivers; other factors include the norms of the society and culture in which we live, religious or spiritual beliefs we may hold, the influence of our peers, as well as the time in history and world events that have occurred or are currently happening. All these elements combine to make us into the adults we will become and impact our reproductive story. The following are some examples of the way various dynamics and experiences can affect us.

Take, for instance, Andrea, whose father suddenly passed away when she was 14 years old. Andrea offered the following:

> My household went from relative calm to utter chaos. My mother was so depressed, had to take on another job, and relied on me to take care of my two younger brothers. School became a sanctuary for me where I could just concentrate on learning, because when

> I came home, I had to cook dinner, make sure my brothers did their homework, get them to bed—basically I became an adult overnight. I was so torn—wanting to escape and go away to college, yet feeling guilty about leaving. I think it has made me not want to rush into having kids myself, if I want them at all.

The impact that her father's death had on the dynamics in her family had a profound effect on Andrea's desire to have children.

Some people may feel pressure to have children at a certain time, depending on the norms of the culture they are raised in. For example, many migrants of Arab descent in the United States are expected to have children immediately after they marry (Grocher & Gerrits, 2023). Perhaps all your friends got married and started having kids right out of high school. It is natural that you would be influenced by this expectation; it is very common to want to have children when our friends do. As we will discuss, it can be devastating when friends are starting their families and you are struggling to do so.

Other people may delay their desire to have children because of educational pursuits. Stephanie and Eugene, both pursuing careers in medicine, knew they wanted children someday, but they wanted to wait until they had completed their training. People with higher degrees of education tend to delay childbearing, which might increase their risk of miscarriage and age-related infertility (Matthews & Ventura, 1997). If you started a family at an older age, you may feel guilt and question past decisions. This too will be addressed in subsequent chapters.

For many, it is financial insecurity that influences their parenting timeline. Jack and his wife, Lisa, are currently living with his parents. Jack said,

> It is the best choice for now. Student loans are daunting, and we want kids sooner rather than later. Never mind buying a home, we can't even afford to rent something. Living with my parents is not ideal, but it will allow us to get some solid footing under us.

Jack and Lisa both have decent-paying jobs but did not anticipate that wanting to start a family would be impacted by the high cost of living. Their story had to morph to include the realities of their current economic situation. How we manage and cope with unanticipated life situations—be they economic or otherwise—is key to making decisions about starting a family.

Another external factor shaping peoples' reproductive stories today has to do with climate change. A survey was done with students aged 18 to 35, the typical range for individuals who are of or approaching childbearing age (Schwartz et al., 2022). Participants expressed deep concerns about bringing kids into a world where their future might be at risk because of the unprecedented extreme climate events we witness all too frequently. Some in the study thought they might not want to have children, so as not to contribute to overpopulation and global warming and thereby help our planet survive (Schwartz et al., 2022). The times we are living in and changes in weather patterns are very unsettling. Predictions of extreme heat, unprecedented fires, and floods of biblical proportions around the world seem to be in the news daily. How we grapple with our personal desires for children and worries over the future of the world is no doubt challenging and anxiety provoking.

Whatever may have factored into your reproductive story, it is helpful to reflect on how your thoughts and feelings about parenthood have changed over the course of your life. Gaining insight allows you to see what having a family means to you, as well as the impact on your life when a reproductive loss occurs. What you thought your story would look like may have changed because of life's circumstances, but it likely did not include difficulties in trying to have a baby. Although it is not easy, you may be able to cope with many of the snags and complications of life; yet the loss of a hoped-for baby is a trauma that hits at your very core.

THE CHAPTER YOU ARE IN NOW

It is important to remember that this reproductive storyline—beginning in early childhood and morphing as you have matured—is so deeply ingrained that it is an integral part of you. The reproductive story is a fundamental piece of your identity, even if you have not been consciously aware of it. Often, it is only when you have experienced a reproductive loss or trauma that you become aware of the story that was there all along. The expectations that you may have had—that everyone can have a baby, that you can have one when you choose, that you are healthy and strong, or that it is bound to happen if you just keep trying—may blow apart in an instant.

The space you are now in includes the obvious loss of the pregnancy and your baby. With that, you may be experiencing many other wounds as well. Understanding the depth of your multiple losses can help make sense of this crisis. A pregnancy loss affects how you feel about yourself and your self-esteem. It also impacts your relationships—not only with your partner but also with family and friends. And then there is coping with exposure to the rest of the world, where it can seem that everyone is either pregnant or has an infant in their arms. As we walk through these losses in the following sections, you may find that some hit home but others do not, and that's okay. We are not all put together the same way. It can be helpful, however, to understand the multiple layers of loss that can occur and why you are feeling so distraught and confused.

I Feel Like I Have Lost Myself

The loss of self-worth is often one of the first things people talk about when they come in for therapy. Any feelings of insecurity that you may have had about yourself, your competence, or your relationships become heightened with a pregnancy loss or infertility.

Becoming pregnant, in fact, may have made you feel more powerful and sure of yourself. It may have boosted your sense of self as a woman. Likewise, it can make men feel more potent and vital. The internal strivings and development of your parental identity over all the years finally came to fruition.

When infertility or a pregnancy loss occurs, your self-esteem may be stressed. You may even ask yourself, "What is the purpose of my life?" You may wonder if your partner would be better off leaving you so that they could have children with someone else. These are horrible feelings to have, but you are not alone in having them. You may feel alone, frightened, depressed, and insecure, and you may not know which way to turn. Your partner, the very person who may be your go-to in times of distress, is likely going through their own struggles and may not be emotionally available to you. Other people who usually support you—your parents, siblings, or friends—are often at a loss as to what to do or say.

When you begin your journey to becoming a parent, your identity shifts from taking care of yourself to taking care of another human. Even if you have fantasized about it for years, you become a different person when the reality of that change hits. This is what the third separation/individuation phase is all about (Colarusso, 1990). You change with the added layer of responsibility. You grow as you see the world through the eyes of a child. You get to see your own childhood through a different lens and gain a new perspective on life.

With fertility struggles or a pregnancy loss, however, a piece of yourself—quite literally—is taken away. Of course, there are many facets to who you are: You have a work life and a home life. You have friends and colleagues and are part of a community. The loss of a baby or a hoped-for baby, however, reduces all those many sides of you to rubble and ruins. You may find it impossible—at least at first—to find that vibrant, loving, lovable part of you. It is so hard to pick up the pieces of your life when you are feeling so empty.

Although the possibility for growth feels as if it no longer exists, you need to remember that it does. As we will discuss later, finding meaning again—and with it, hope—is an important and attainable goal whether you are able to have children or not.

My Body Isn't Working Right

One assumption about pregnancy is that it is something that everyone can achieve if they want to. This is not always the case. Getting pregnant and staying pregnant is not a guarantee. In fact, the idea that a woman's body can grow another human being is miraculous and is nothing to take for granted. All the pieces of the puzzle must come together for a pregnancy to be successful and result in a healthy live birth—and they usually do. That is the miracle. Unfortunately, as you (or your loved one) have experienced, this is not always the case.

The shame that overtakes people who are struggling with fertility issues, have had a pregnancy loss, had to terminate a pregnancy for medical reasons, or experienced the death of a newborn can be overwhelming. You may ask yourself, "What did I do wrong?" Self-blame is so common in these cases. Often, I have heard women say their womb was not a safe place for their baby. You may feel defective and flawed. Searching for a reason to explain this loss is normal. Sometimes reasons can be found—perhaps the umbilical cord was too long, and your baby's oxygen supply was cut off—but this is not a reflection of anything you did or did not do. It has to do with the way the pregnancy developed. It can be hard to appreciate that this is a system unto itself, which you do not have control over.

Having control over situations, as well as having control over your own body, is a fundamental and universal desire. When I think about how a baby develops—from the early divisions of cells to the structuring of the brain, the limbs, and all the internal organs—it is with a sense of awe that a woman's body knows how to do this. All of this goes on without our awareness. Yet when something goes wrong, it can feel as if we are responsible. We try to take control and find answers.

Sometimes there just aren't any reasons that we know of for the loss. Accepting this can be very difficult. Wanting to fix the problem is only natural; if you could correct the problem by either doing or not doing something and change a future outcome, then that would be the best outcome. The frustration of knowing there was nothing you could have done differently and there is nothing you can do to prevent a future loss can feel overwhelming. One thing to remember is that every pregnancy is different. It is natural to worry that the same loss will occur if or when you get pregnant again, but just because you have had a previous loss does not necessarily mean that the next pregnancy will have the same outcome. In fact, if you have had a single miscarriage, it may be helpful to know that at least 85% of women go on to have a successful pregnancy when they try again (American Pregnancy Association, 2024). Even if you have had two or three losses, it may also be helpful to consider that 75% of women go on to have a healthy pregnancy (American Pregnancy Association, 2024).

What's Happening to My Relationship?

We all want to be understood. Many times, when I work with reproductive clients, they want to know whether I "get it." That is, do I get the nightmare and pain of this kind of loss? Sometimes people will ask me personal questions about my own reproductive history. Over the years, I have come to see these questions not so much as a desire to know my story but as a craving for understanding: "Will you be able to help me, or will you think of this loss as something insignificant?" Of course, we may turn to our partners for understanding as well. What happens, though, if you and your partner find yourselves unable to support each other? What happens when the person you feel closest to suddenly feels like a stranger or, worse, an enemy?

Whether you are in a same-sex or heterosexual relationship, you and your partner have gone through this loss together, but you may each be experiencing it differently. Not only do you both have your own reproductive story, but you each also have your own unique ways of grieving and coping. In Chapter 4, we'll discuss the process of grieving a reproductive loss in detail, but suffice it to say that what looks like grief to one person may not be the same for another. Some people need to cry and withdraw, while others need to throw themselves back into work and activities. Some people need to talk about what happened, while others need not to talk about it. These two seemingly opposite reactions are both consequences of the loss, and both are valid ways of grieving.

Complicating matters further, both you and your partner may manage your grief differently from moment to moment. Grief has no specific timeline. One of you may want to numb your feelings at a particular time by spacing out in front of the TV, while the other may need to engage and talk about their feelings—and these two modes of being can flip-flop repeatedly. Meeting each other at the same point is challenging. Misunderstandings may grow. If it feels like your partner isn't with you, it doesn't mean that your relationship is falling apart—it just means that you are both in your own corners trying to figure out how to help yourself and help each other through this impossible grief.

Be patient and be gentle with each other. The person you hold dear is going through a very hard time—as are you. There is a natural tendency to want to fix it for each other, but for some things, such as a pregnancy loss and the grief that follows, fixing takes time. Couple's therapy may be something that you consider. Being in therapy together ensures a dedicated time for both of you to focus on the loss and on any issues that may erupt because of it. It can allow you to plan—together—for those moments when you can't engage. Knowing that you will be able to come together in therapy may make it easier to give each other time and space apart. Women tend to seek out psychological services more than men do, but men will often come to therapy when they think it will help their partner through this tough time (Nam et al., 2010).

Sex? I'm Not Sure I'm Ready

One of the things couples struggle with following a pregnancy loss is sexual intimacy. It may be the last thing on your mind. Depending on the loss that has occurred (e.g., a miscarriage, an ectopic pregnancy, or a stillbirth), you may need to wait until your body heals and you feel better—both physically and emotionally. After a miscarriage, you can probably resume sexual relations after your bleeding stops, but you may not want to. There is a difference between being physically cleared to have sex (and this is something you should definitely discuss with your doctor) and being mentally prepared. Your body may heal faster than the emotional wounds do. For some, sexual intimacy can feel like a reminder of the loss and trigger a host of negative feelings. Sex can bring up fears about getting pregnant again—even though that may be the goal. The anxiety about another pregnancy loss, which we'll talk more about in Chapter 7, is real. The important thing is for you and your partner to take the time you need to grieve and work through your feelings.

What if your partner is ready and you are not? This is a common occurrence and can lead to more strain and misunderstanding in your relationship. If you are not yet ready but your partner is, they may feel hurt and rejected by a flat-out "no." Talking with each other about your feelings is key. Finding other ways to share physical closeness—cuddling, holding hands, hugging—may help you reassure each other that you are still connected.

Where Do We Fit In?

Maddie and Sam have a wide network of friends, many of whom have either just had their first baby or are pregnant. They were so excited when her pregnancy test was positive; they were now official members of "the club," as they said. It was a hot day when they went in for a routine ultrasound appointment. They were shocked to learn that their baby had no heartbeat. Maddie described what happened:

> I was already sweating from the heat outside when I laid down on the exam table, but then when I saw the sonographer's face I started sweating even more. I knew instantly that something was wrong by her crestfallen look. One minute we were all chatting, it was very upbeat, and the next it was like a dark cloud came over her face. That sinking feeling, I felt so sick to my stomach, and even before anything was confirmed I was sobbing.

Sam looked as if he had seen a ghost. He described what he was feeling in that moment:

> It was like something in me snapped. I remember feeling icy cold in spite of the hot weather, scared, and panicked that I couldn't stop what was happening. I know I squeezed Maddie's hand, but what I really wanted to do was grab that damn monitor and hurl it across the room. I will never forget that moment.

Both Maddie and Sam were in shock. As the news of their loss sunk in, they faced the arduous task of letting everyone know. They were not only shaken by how people reacted, as we'll discuss in the following subsection, but their grief also was intensified by feeling set apart and different from their peers. Would they be able to maintain their relationships with their friends who were pregnant or new parents? Sam stated:

> Suddenly we felt ousted. Not that our friends didn't include us, but we didn't want to bring everyone down. We just couldn't

> relate anymore. Talk about diapers, sleep schedules, tummy time—which we had been excited about before—no longer made any sense. In fact, it only filled me with rage—a silent rage, of course I would never do anything—but I felt angry to my core. We've really pulled back, and we're not sure where we fit in anymore.

Not only did Maddie and Sam feel out of place with this set of friends who were focused on parenting, but they also were struggling to feel connected with friends whose thoughts of becoming parents were either way off in the future or nonexistent. That is because Maddie and Sam became *psychological parents*; they transitioned into a new developmental phase even though they had a pregnancy loss (Jaffe & Diamond, 2011). As Maddie noted, "It feels awkward to be with these other sets of friends as well. They're sympathetic, but they really don't know what to do or say." Caught in a limbo state, Maddie and Sam felt isolated and alone.

Maddie and Sam are parents in their hearts and minds, but they do not have a living child to prove it. This is such a common feeling for people who have had a pregnancy loss. Admission into the so-called club with full membership privileges has been taken away. So many patients I have worked with in this situation struggle when asked about children. How do you answer a question such as "Do you have any kids?" or "How many kids do you have?" Do you let others know that you have lost a child? If you have living children, do you say, "Yes, I have two children. One is living, and one is not"? Or is it better to say, "I have one kid"? Many people worry that they are dishonoring the child who has passed if they don't talk about it, while others are concerned about bringing up a very painful subject in a social milieu. These are moment-to-moment decisions, depending on the situation and how you are feeling at that time. Sometimes people give one answer outwardly but think the true answer to themselves.

My Friends and Family Don't Know What to Say

Maddie and Sam are not the only people to express their feelings of isolation and awkwardness. While your close friends and family want to be there for you, they might not know how. In their effort to support and soothe you, they might say things that are more off-putting than helpful, making the situation worse. You have probably heard statements like these: "Don't worry, you'll be able to have another," "It was for the best," or "Just relax and it will happen." You might be able to have another pregnancy and child, but that cannot replace the child you lost. And clearly, having a pregnancy loss or fertility struggles is not "for the best"; what would be best is to have a healthy pregnancy and baby.

When people make these kinds of statements, it is likely that they are feeling unnerved by your loss. They may be unsure of whether to talk about it with you at all—this can be awkward, to say the least. If they avoid talking about it, you probably feel invisible and discounted. You've experienced a trauma unlike any other, and not to have it recognized is unsettling and hurtful. If people do address your loss and make remarks that are off-putting, you need to decide how to handle it. Perhaps you just smile and let it go, understanding their intentions. Or you may want to let them know that their comments are not helpful and, in fact, are just the opposite. How do you do so and not completely alienate them?

It may help to think that these individuals are trying their best; they are hurting for you. No one really knows how to handle themselves when addressing pregnancy loss or infertility. You may find yourself in the odd position of needing to comfort them. They may turn to you for guidance on what to say or do. You can use this as an opportunity to teach people what you need by letting them know that a simple statement, such as "I am so sorry for your loss," can provide the most comfort.

It can be helpful to have some ready retorts on hand to protect yourself from others' well-meaning but painful comments. For example, upon learning about Gwen's miscarriage, Gwen's mother-in-law Adele said, "Well, at least it was early. It would be worse if you had felt the baby moving." Gwen, who had always had an open relationship with Adele, was deeply hurt by that comment. She realized Adele had no idea how deeply her remark stung. Gwen gently gave Adele some feedback: "I know you are just trying to make me feel better, but it doesn't matter how long I had been pregnant. We lost our baby; he was so very much wanted and loved, whether I felt him moving or not." Gwen went on to talk about her reproductive story and all the hopes and dreams she had for this baby. Taking this as an opportunity, Gwen was able to help Adele understand the depth and meaning of this traumatic event.

Grandparents-to-be have their own struggles as they observe the grief of their adult children. Just like Adele, your parents may try to make you feel better but say or do the wrong thing in the process. We know that grandparents too have a reproductive story, and their loss is multilayered. Their fantasies about helping to nurture, support, and care for a grandchild have been dashed. Not only that, they also are witnesses to your pain. They may be trying to protect you, their child, from feelings of grief and loss. They may be wrestling with their own history of pregnancy and birth—whether that included a loss or not. Sometimes grandparents feel guilty about their own fertility or ease at having children and cannot imagine the depth of your pain. As with Gwen, you may be in a position of having to educate your parents or your partner's parents about what it is that you need.

Seeing Other Pregnant Women: When Nowhere Feels Safe

"They are everywhere!" cried Lena. "I can't seem to go anywhere without spying a baby bump!" Adding to the trauma of your pregnancy loss is the worry about being triggered whenever you engage with people. For example, a friend may announce she's pregnant. A baby shower for a colleague may be held at your place of work. You may need to go back to your doctor's office for follow-ups, and other pregnant women may be sitting in the waiting room. This feeling that the only safe place is at home is yet another element that adds to your loss. Even then, you may turn on the news or watch a movie, and someone in the story is pregnant. As you cautiously step out into the world, you may find emotional land mines at every turn.

Learning how to protect yourself from being overwhelmed by these triggers is key. Attending a gathering may sound wonderful at one moment, and the next you may feel like shuttering yourself up in a dark room and never going out again. Is it okay to skip a friend's baby shower? Absolutely. Depending on the friend, being open about your feelings—that you are just not able to celebrate with her in a group situation—is a way of taking care of yourself. You can let your friend know that you would love to get together privately. If you feel you must attend, another strategy is to go late and leave early. This strategy applies to all social engagements—even those with your family. You may find it especially difficult around holidays. So many family traditions are focused on children, and it might be just too much to deal with right now.

Apart from moving to a deserted island, you will be exposed to the child-centric world we live in. Learning how to cope with the challenges of navigating a path forward is discussed more in Chapter 6. The rug that we talked about in Chapter 1—that metaphor for order and stability—has been yanked out from under you, with all your feelings of normalcy flying around in the air. Until things have settled, you will likely feel off kilter. Most important is to take care of yourself and each other.

RECONSTRUCTING YOUR STORY AFTER YOUR LOSS

These multiple layers of loss—losing confidence in yourself, having difficulties in your relationship, struggling in social interactions, and feeling retriggered at every turn—can be encapsulated and understood by the loss of your hoped-for reproductive story. It is this story that connects you to your unborn child. When the story unravels, the emotional injury you feel is equal to the attachment and love you have for your baby. Pregnancy loss upends it all. You are in a crisis that hits at your very core. You may question everything: "Why is this happening? Can I go on? Did I do something to deserve this? What is wrong with me?" The world may no longer feel like a safe place; you may feel that you are out of step, no longer fitting in the way you did before. The jolt to your system and your sense of self can be shocking. You may feel depressed, anxious, traumatized, and scared. It is so important to remember this: These are normal responses to this devastating situation. How could you possibly feel like your old self when the worst has occurred? The current chapter of the story you are in has been disrupted and with it the very foundation of your beliefs, your hopes, and your expectations.

Perhaps it would help to think about the reproductive story as a house. You have built it from the bottom up over time, piece by piece starting from your childhood, using good materials and providing it with as strong a foundation as you could. You have lovingly placed cabinets and bookshelves and designed it to be comfortable and cozy. But just as you are ready to add another floor to the construction, an earthquake occurs. The beams crack, there are holes in the flooring, and the windows break.

The house is a metaphor for you and creating a family. Right now, everything has been shattered. It may feel as if you will never be able to rebuild. Let's think, though, how you might be able to reconstruct your house. You may have to tear down some walls to build new ones. You may have to haul off some debris to clear space.

You may also need to just sit and stare at the devastation before you can make a new plan. This is hard work: It cannot be done alone or quickly, but it can be done.

You may not be able to imagine that you can rebuild right now. Allowing yourself time to grieve is necessary in the process of building a new structure. Learning coping strategies to interact with people who may not fully understand can be likened to buying new tools to help with the construction. Engaging with people who can help support you is vital. Restructuring the overall design can open pathways and plans that you hadn't thought of before. It also may be that the reconstruction does not proceed in an even manner: You may do some construction, but then need to take a step back and just sit and stare again. This is a common process in grieving—as they say, two steps forward and one back.

In Greek mythology, the phoenix is an immortal bird. It is reborn again and again out of the ashes of a phoenix that has died. The symbolic message is one of renewal. Indeed, out of trauma and despair, growth can occur. As mentioned in the Introduction of this volume, the term *posttraumatic growth* refers to the potential for positive change in a person's life when a trauma occurs (Tedeschi & Calhoun, 2004). We'll talk about this much more in Chapter 8, but first steps first. This is the time to grieve. Exercise 2.2 entails looking at your story before your loss and looking at it now.

EXERCISE 2.2. Your Story Then, Your Story Now

Whatever your pregnancy loss, the meaning of it is unique to you and your situation. Your story has gone awry and, right now, you may feel like it will never get on track again. You may not have even realized that you had a reproductive story until your loss.

(*continues*)

EXERCISE 2.2. Your Story Then, Your Story Now (*Continued*)

A helpful first step is to write down your original story in as much detail as possible. Include all the fantasies you may have had about becoming a parent someday. If writing isn't something you like to do, then maybe tell your story to someone close to you. Perhaps you and your partner, if you have one, can do this exercise together and share your stories with each other.

Then let's work on the story of your loss. Writing and sharing this part of the story is an important step in the healing process. Sometimes just getting the words out stops them from incessantly swirling in your head. Telling the story of your loss is kind of like taking out a splinter. If you don't remove it, it will fester and get infected. The same thing is true with our emotions. If we keep them bottled up inside, they get bigger and bigger until it feels like they will explode. Even if it hurts to get them out, just like it does with a splinter, telling our story allows us to heal.

When clients in psychotherapy tell me their stories, no detail is too small or insignificant. Examples can include the sounds and smells in the room, the look on someone's face, the fluorescent lights of an emergency room, and so on. You might remember feeling physical pain or seeing blood. People might give you this advice: "Don't dwell on it. Put it behind you and move forward." What I am suggesting, however, is just the opposite. As much as you may want to push all of this away, it is the deliberate attention to the specifics of your loss that can make you feel more in control. Addressing all the details of how your story went off course is the emotional equivalent of removing a splinter.

Each time you tell your story, it will be a different experience and you will learn from it. It changes over time. Some details may become more salient, while others fade into the background. It also may differ depending on who is listening and their response. Perhaps in telling someone your story, they will tell you their story or share their perspective. Growth and change come from getting support from others who you can trust and feel safe with. As a first step, this exercise will allow you to see just how far away from your original fantasy and dreams of parenthood your story has gone. Understanding what you have lost—some combination of your identity, your relationships with others, and your future—verifies that this is not something to minimize. Giving voice to your feelings is vital to healing.

SUMMARY

From early childhood onward, the reproductive story is embedded into our very core. We may be aware of it at times, but often it grows and develops as we do, buried in our unconscious. It is often only when we are confronted with the trauma of pregnancy loss that we recognize how significant it is to become a parent. The meaning and importance of the story becomes evident as we struggle with healing and reconstructing our lives.

Reproductive losses of all kinds can be considered traumatic. In Chapter 3, we will define trauma from different perspectives, and we will focus on what happens when deeply held assumptions about life and pregnancy are disrupted. The more you are able to understand this trauma and loss, the more you will be able to grieve and find a path forward.

CHAPTER 3

THE TRAUMA OF A PREGNANCY LOSS: WHAT HAPPENS WHEN DREAMS ARE SHATTERED?

Pregnancy loss is a medical trauma as well as a psychological one. In this chapter, we'll explore how mental health professionals define trauma; doing so will help you understand your own traumatic experience. As described in Chapter 2, it is not just the loss of your pregnancy that you are coping with, but it is also the loss of your reproductive story and the multiple areas of your life that it has impacted. Previous traumas, events from your past that you may have worked through and resolved, may suddenly rear up again. You may be feeling okay, and then seemingly out of the blue, something triggers you and your emotions feel like they are soaring out of control. Research suggests that we all have fundamental assumptions about life—these are benevolence, predictability, and control (Tedeschi & Calhoun, 2004). As we will learn in this chapter, these assumptions (also referred to as *core beliefs*) may be shattered by reproductive loss. Ultimately, being able to pick up the shattered pieces, reflect on the trauma of pregnancy loss, and rewrite your story will help you heal.

WHAT IS TRAUMA?

You may know about the *DSM*, or the *Diagnostic and Statistical Manual of Mental Disorders*. It's what mental health professionals think of as their bible; we rely on it to help analyze symptoms, understand patterns of behavior, and diagnose patients. We use it to formulate how best to treat a patient. For example, the *DSM* diagnostic criteria for posttraumatic stress disorder (PTSD) define *trauma* as "exposure to actual or threatened death, serious injury, or sexual violence" (American Psychiatric Association, 2022, p. 301). The exposure can happen to you directly or to someone who has witnessed the event. You can also be traumatized if you learn that someone close to you—a family member or friend—has experienced a trauma. This kind of exposure brings on feelings of distress, with mood fluctuations.

People with PTSD may react with intensified anxiety or depression; others may feel both. Many people suffer from intrusive thoughts and memories, with flashbacks—a kind of disturbing reliving—of the event. It is not uncommon for people to have sleep disturbances from both ends of the spectrum (either wanting to sleep all the time or experiencing insomnia), and they may attempt to avoid all reminders of the event, withdrawing from interactions with others. Some people can become agitated, while others feel numb. Whatever one's reaction, we often think of PTSD as happening after a one-time occurrence, such as an earthquake, a school shooting, or a car accident. But PTSD can also be chronic; we see it in soldiers who go into battle over and over. We also see it in people witnessing or living through the effects of poverty and in caregivers working in a hospital with daily exposure to illness and death.

Many people who have experienced a pregnancy loss may be diagnosed with PTSD. One-time events such as an ectopic pregnancy, a stillbirth, a termination for a medical reason, or a miscarriage can readily fall under this category. Likewise, people who experience the chronicity of infertility, multiple miscarriages, or failed medical interventions such as in vitro fertilization (IVF) can also receive a psychological diagnosis of PTSD. Sadly, many people experience both—for example, they suffer a one-time event such as a miscarriage and are also coping with ongoing fertility struggles. A study was conducted with nearly 3,000 childless women who experienced a pregnancy loss, infertility, or both (Schwerdtfeger & Shreffler, 2009). The researchers found high levels of depression and low levels of life satisfaction in both groups. Not surprisingly, the women who experienced both pregnancy loss and fertility issues reported the highest levels of distress.

Not everyone, however, who has suffered a pregnancy loss, infertility, or both has symptoms that meet the diagnostic criteria for PTSD. Sometimes people can have some symptoms of PTSD but they may not fit all the categories and descriptors set forth in the *DSM*. Just because your symptoms don't fit the diagnostic criteria does not mean that you haven't suffered a trauma. There is another definition of trauma—somewhat broader in scope—that may better illustrate what you have experienced. This definition describes trauma as an event (or events) that causes the disintegration of your inner world, how you think about yourself, what you hope for, and your life (Cann et al., 2010). This event can overwhelmingly shatter your core beliefs and assumptions. When your pregnancy has not gone as you anticipated, thoughts and feelings about yourself, your relationships, and your life can change in profound ways.

CORE BELIEFS: BENEVOLENCE, PREDICTABILITY, AND CONTROL

So, what are core beliefs and assumptions? As noted earlier, research has pointed to three primary ideas that we all hold to be true: benevolence, predictability, and control (Tedeschi & Calhoun, 2004). Let's look at each of these concepts and see how they apply to people in a general sense. Then we can examine them to see what happens when they are undone by reproductive events.

Benevolence refers to the overriding feeling that the world is a good place, filled with kind and caring people. Even if we know on some level that this is not true, we want to believe it is. Benevolence allows us to form bonds with people. We can trust them and create a sense of mutual interdependence. During the height of the COVID-19 pandemic, I was pleasantly surprised by my wonderful neighbors. We all made ourselves available to each other—checking in to see who needed what when one of us went to the store, making sure that everyone was safe. That's an example of benevolence. We can also think about things we may take for granted, such as hiring a mechanic to fix our car. We trust that they have the training and skills to get the job done. We are leaving them with a very valuable piece of property, with the belief that they know how to repair the car and it will then be safe to drive. The car shop needs to trust that we will pay them for their work. The system works because of trust and belief in one another. You can imagine that without this mutual sense of dependence—the belief in benevolence—chaos could ensue.

Predictability refers to the consistency and structure of our lives. We take comfort in knowing what to expect, making plans, and following through on them. Think about your daily routine: The alarm goes off, the coffee pot goes on, and you ready yourself for the day. For most of us, yesterday was pretty much like today, and today will be pretty much like tomorrow. There may be different things on the to-do list, but the overall rhythm of each day will likely be the same. Even if we complain about the grind of our daily routine, people generally like this kind of regularity. It brings comfort. We also take comfort in the patterns of a year; we forecast the seasons and celebrate the holidays, with one naturally following another. Predictability is not only about the course of a day or year, but it also refers to the expectations of a lifetime. We anticipate that children will become adults, have careers and families of their own, grow old, and eventually die.

Control is that core belief that strives to feel in charge. It is that feeling of mastery, of knowing "I've got this!" When we know we have the skills to handle something—or any number of situations—we feel empowered. If or when things feel out of control, and they often do, there is a natural impulse to find a way to regulate or manage the situation. Think about an accident that may have occurred, such as a car running into a telephone pole. Clearly, the driver lost control. We feel concern for the people in the car; at the same time, we may wonder what caused the accident. Did the driver fall asleep at the wheel? Were they inebriated? Was there something wrong with the car? Our effort to find reasons for events is an attempt to stay in control. We can then try to make sure that none of these things will occur when we are driving. It is much more difficult to believe that random events can happen for no reason, as they often do when we consider pregnancy loss.

WHEN ASSUMPTIONS ARE SHATTERED

Consider this situation: You are watching children play outdoors in front of your house when an errant baseball accidentally smashes through your living room window. There are shards of glass everywhere—what had been whole is now scattered into small and dangerous pieces. How do you handle the situation? When you look out the window, you see some kids are running away in fear, others are standing there in shock and guilt, and still others are in tears. You are probably feeling annoyed, but perhaps at the same time you also understand that accidents happen. Yes, this creates a hassle for you: You need to clean up the mess and find someone to replace the window. You may also have empathy for the kids, knowing that the window break wasn't intentional. All these emotions—yours and the kids—are released with the shattering of a piece of glass.

Now imagine that it's not a window that has been broken, but it is your pregnancy or attempt at pregnancy that has failed. Just like the kids, you may want to run away and avoid the reality of the situation. No doubt you are in shock. Trying to make sense of it all, you may blame yourself and feel guilty about something you think you did wrong to deserve this. You may feel despondent and hopeless. Your sense of self—of feeling competent and in control—is shattered. Cleaning this up is not as simple as picking up pieces of glass and vacuuming the room. There is no fix-it person who can put things back to normal. With a broken window, you know just what to do; with a pregnancy loss and feeling broken yourself, what comes next may not be very clear.

Figure 3.1 illustrates many of the emotions that can happen when a pregnancy loss occurs. Imagine each as a slice of broken window glass—if not handled with care, more pain gets inflicted. Underlying all of these emotions is the shattering of your basic core assumptions of a just, fair, and predictable world.

With the shattering of the basic core beliefs of benevolence, predictability, and control, it is no wonder that your feelings are all

FIGURE 3.1. Emotional Reactions When Pregnancy Dreams Are Shattered

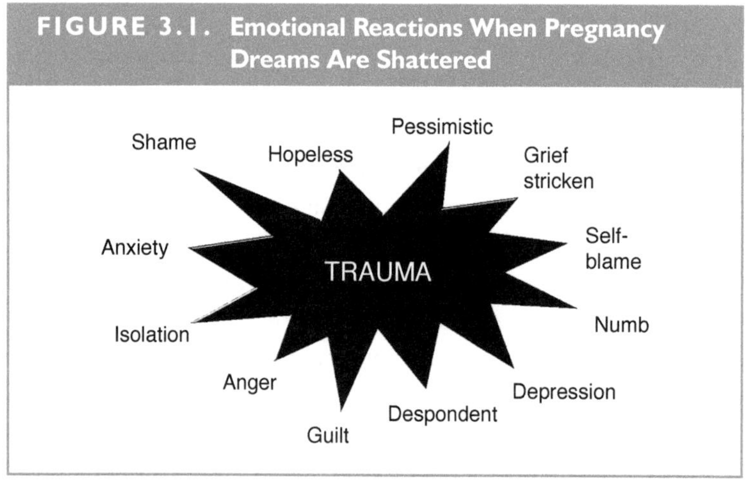

over the place. Researchers have compared this to an earthquake, stating that it is "a psychologically seismic event that can severely shake, threaten, or reduce to rubble" the structures that have guided you through life (Tedeschi & Calhoun, 2004, p. 5). You may feel like you are floundering, you cannot make any decisions, and what was once meaningful is no more. You have been traumatized and may feel that you have lost your way.

WHAT ARE CORE BELIEFS ABOUT PREGNANCY?

Knowing about general core beliefs helps us consider the fundamental beliefs you may have about pregnancy, childbirth, and parenting. In this section, we'll discuss many assumptions people have about pregnancy and what happens when these assumptions are destroyed. As you read through this section, you may find that some beliefs resonate with you more than others; it may also make you think about other beliefs you have had about pregnancy that are not listed here. The point is to help you understand what you thought about before your loss and how you feel now. Understanding your loss from this perspective and recognizing how deeply ingrained these basic beliefs are can facilitate the healing process. The more you understand yourself and what is wrong, the more you can—metaphorically—pick up the broken glass and install a new window.

Core Belief 1: I Am Strong and Healthy

Meet Alicia, a 31-year-old woman of Mexican and White descent. She is a physical therapist, is constantly on the go, and wears her long black hair in a messy bun to keep it out of her way. In our session, Alicia described her work this way: "I work with people of all ages every day, helping them heal from physical injuries. It's so gratifying to see people gain their full range of motion and gain their strength back." She went on to talk about her pregnancy:

> Prior to getting pregnant, I wanted to be in the best shape I could. I put myself on a schedule of strength building exercises, yoga, and aerobics. I thought the stronger I was, the easier it would be to manage all that pregnancy weight and carry it.

She sighed, "Well, we know how great that went." Alicia experienced a miscarriage at 10 weeks, despite all her good intentions. "I never would have thought this would happen to me," she said.

If you are of reproductive age, you are most likely in the prime of your life, and you, like Alicia, may be healthy and strong. You may pride yourself on working out and taking care of your body, or you may have "exercise more" on your to-do list. Regardless, you may not have considered pregnancy as something that would be physically challenging or would not work out the way you expected. Because we think about pregnancy as something that is natural, there is a common belief that anyone who wants to have a baby should be able to do so, especially if she is young and healthy.

While the odds are in your favor of pregnancy and childbirth happening without trauma, we know it is not a given. There is no predicting the course of a pregnancy if, in fact, a woman can conceive at all. There are so many things that need to go right, so many ways that a fetus must develop correctly—it truly is a miracle when everything works as it should. When a pregnancy doesn't happen as anticipated, you may no longer feel healthy and strong. You may find yourself suddenly thrust into the medical world and feel diseased and physically impaired. Even the way the Practice Committee of the American Society for Reproductive Medicine (2023) describes infertility falls into the disease model: "Infertility is a disease, condition, or status characterized by . . . the inability to achieve a successful pregnancy based on a patient's medical, sexual, and reproductive history, age, physical findings, diagnostic testing, or any combination of those factors."

Pregnancy can be very demanding physically. The hormonal changes that produce symptoms of nausea, fatigue, breast tenderness, lightheadedness, and brain fog are all normal and anticipated reactions. Other bodily changes, however, may be warnings that things are not going well. The pain that accompanies an ectopic pregnancy, for example, needs to be addressed immediately. Likewise, high blood pressure is an indicator of preeclampsia, which can lead to preterm labor and be lethal for the mother if untreated. It can be absolutely crushing to have a pregnancy demise and then have breast milk come in without a baby to feed. Your body may be continuing to act as it should after giving birth, but nothing feels normal about it. Indeed, it can feel as if your body is betraying you.

This shift in how you see yourself—from healthy to diseased—is significant. As Alicia, the physical therapist we discussed earlier, put it, "My work is focused on getting people's bodies out of disease and back to health. But there is nothing I can do for myself. There is no physical therapy to fix a miscarriage." The loss of seeing oneself as healthy can prove to be a major blow to one's self-esteem. Many reproductive traumas land women in the hospital; in fact, this may be the first medical crisis you have had to face in your life. As another woman described it,

> I felt my identity slip away when I put on that flimsy hospital gown. I was no longer "me;" I morphed into "a patient" who got a medical bracelet and number. None of my accomplishments mattered; I was just a body on someone's workload.

Many feelings accompany this medical upheaval, ranging from feeling incompetent ("My body has let me down"), to diminished ("I am worthless"), to frightened ("What is going to happen next?"). Think back to the basic core beliefs and it can feel as if they have all been altered. The world has stopped feeling like a safe place where things are in your control and you know what to expect. That which you could count on—your strong body and good health—may feel greatly diminished.

Core Belief 2: My Peers and I Would All Have Kids at the Same Time

Kara described the social struggles that she and her husband, Jonathan, were experiencing:

> A few years back, everyone I knew was getting married. One year, Jonathan and I went to six weddings! We felt part of this group, as we too got married 3 years ago. Now all our friends are starting to have kids; some are even pregnant with their second child. We feel out of the loop, out of sync. We don't feel as if we fit in anymore.

If you feel left behind on the assumptive timeline to have children, it can add to the feelings of trauma and loss. Everyone else seems to be in another chapter—moving forward with their lives—while you feel stuck. It's as if you have been invited to a dinner party and all the other adults are sitting at the adult table while you are still being seated with the kids.

From a psychological view, an interesting development takes place when people decide to have children. A shift happens in one's identity as the reality of becoming a parent takes shape. You move from thinking about your own needs to thinking about the needs of a baby as well. These thoughts can happen well before conception occurs. When planning to build a family, it is not uncommon for people to think about their living situation and where they might set up the baby's room. Sometimes they think about buying a new car to fit a car seat more easily; they may have even thought about the schools in the neighborhood and considered moving to a better school district. Once you know you're pregnant, these thoughts intensify. You become a parent psychologically well before you have the goods to prove it.

A pregnancy loss interrupts the cycle in which you would join your friends and family who are having children. Social gatherings may now focus on kids; get-togethers may be dictated by kids' nap schedules. Even when an event is for adults only, talk may veer toward babysitters, day care, preschool, and the like. You may find yourself deciding to spend more time with single friends or couples who are not having kids yet. Even then, you may feel out of place with those relationships as well. You are in limbo: It may be difficult to relate to people who don't have or want children, and it may be just as difficult to relate to people who do.

At the very time when support and understanding is needed, you may want to withdraw from family and friends. That is certainly understandable, but isolating may only cause more distress. A support group may really help (see the Resources in this volume). Whether a group meets in person or online, it can feel like a lifeline and provide information, understanding, and connection. Some groups are geared to a specific type of pregnancy loss or infertility, while others are intended for specific populations (e.g., fathers or grandparents). There are also groups that focus on special issues, such as coping with a subsequent pregnancy or parenting after a loss. Some groups are led by a professional, while others are peer led. You want to make sure that the group provides a safe place where you will be able to tell your story without judgment, learn how others have coped and grieved, and understand that you are not alone.

Core Belief 3: I Am in Control

Years of using birth control and worry over an unplanned pregnancy may have created an illusion that becoming pregnant when you wanted to would be in your control. Perhaps you have thought, as many people do, something like this: "If I get pregnant by such-and-such date, I'll have the baby by the holidays [or in time for summer vacation or another special event]." Consider Barbara, who was hoping to get pregnant and be far enough along so that she could make the announcement at an upcoming family reunion. "I really want to be able to tell everyone in person," she stated. "It would be awesome if I was showing by then and could surprise them all." The idea that a pregnancy can actually be planned disappears with infertility or pregnancy demise. The truth is that conception rarely works on the timetable we would like it to.

It is not just the use of birth control that may give you a sense of being in charge. Self-care in terms of diet, exercise, and sleep hygiene are all attempts at doing the right things for your body and your baby. If your cupboard is filled with junk food, you may decide to toss it and replace it with healthy snacks. Or if you are buying standard apples at the market, for instance, you would not be alone if you opted for the higher-priced organic ones. For many, pregnancy causes an uptick in buying organic products to help ensure the best possible start for the baby by reducing pesticide exposure and increasing nutritional value. Unfortunately, even the best self-care doesn't guarantee that your pregnancy will go as hoped for.

Countless times, I have heard women blame themselves for their pregnancy demise. Here are a few examples of things clients have told me over the years:

- I carried a heavy bag of groceries.
- I pushed myself and stayed late at work.

- It happened right after I ate a bowl of ice cream.
- I was on my feet all day getting the baby's room ready and didn't sit down for a minute.
- I'm sure it was the caffeine in the chocolate cake I ate.
- I shouldn't have mowed the lawn.
- I shouldn't have gone on that long car ride.

One woman, in a heart-wrenching confession, believed that she caused her stillbirth because she wanted to have a boy but she was having a girl. It was important for her to know that her thoughts and feelings could not and did not contribute to the stillbirth.

Unless there is some underlying condition that your doctor is concerned about, the normal activities of a pregnant woman are not responsible for her pregnancy loss. Wanting to find a reason for your loss—even if that reason is flawed—can create a sense of control. Whatever you think caused the loss, you can then be sure not to do it the next time around. The association between what you did (or didn't do) and the loss can be so strong that you may not be able to consider that your reasoning is faulty. It can feel paradoxically better to have some justification for the loss—even if it is not true—than to have no explanation at all. Again, it can provide a much-needed sense of control.

Not feeling in charge—understanding that reproductive events are not within your control—can instill anxiety. You may be told by your medical team that these things happen, that it was not your fault. Even if a loss can be explained medically, you may still believe that you caused it. The rational part of you may understand that you are not at fault; but the emotional side of you may cling to the assumption that it was your body that could not get pregnant or maintain the pregnancy, so you must be to blame.

Core Belief 4: If I Work Hard, I Will Succeed

How many of us were encouraged to persevere after a failure, with the phrase "If at first you don't succeed, try, try again." Another popular adage is "Pull yourself up by your bootstraps." The sentiment around these phrases is well-meaning. They are meant to encourage us not to give up. If you have had a pregnancy loss, you probably do want to try again, but working harder at it may not be possible.

Achieving parenthood is not like studying more to increase your grade point average. Nor is it equivalent to working harder at your job to get a promotion or to reach a deadline. It's also not like exercising more to reach your health goals. Those things are largely in our control; getting and staying pregnant is largely not. This relates back to the fundamental assumption of control. When that core belief is challenged—if you can't work harder at something to make it happen—it can lead to feelings of helplessness and depression.

Some people do try to work harder at getting pregnant—sometimes obsessively. I have witnessed many women spending endless hours on internet research, looking for the best treatment options or the best doctors. You may feel that a change in your diet will do the trick; many women I've worked with have decided to go gluten free. Although there is no definitive research that shows a gluten-free diet will help you get pregnant (unless you have celiac disease; Krawczyk et al., 2022), the hope that it will—or at least the thought that you are trying to approach it differently—may make you feel you've done everything possible to achieve a healthy pregnancy. Men may also strive for changes in lifestyle, diet, and exercise to improve the health of their sperm. Likewise, even after several attempts at IVF, people may want to pursue it one more time—perhaps using a different protocol or going to a different clinic. Many times, people decide to switch doctors after a loss. Sometimes it is just too painful to return to the same medical practice. It may also fuel the belief that you will receive better medical care elsewhere and thereby prevent another loss.

The truth is that getting pregnant or carrying a pregnancy to term is not something you can consciously force your body to do. As stated previously, pregnancy is a complicated biochemical process, which is largely a self-sufficient system. The process of fertilization and fetal development is not something that your thoughts or feelings can control. If it were, then you would be able not to get pregnant simply by just thinking about it. If that were the case, then we could all say goodbye to birth control. If you are someone used to setting goals and achieving them, however, running into the proverbial brick wall of reproductive trauma and loss and not being able to work harder for success can be overwhelming and crushing.

Core Belief 5: Good Things Happen to Good People

We now turn our attention to, of all things, Santa Claus! Regardless of your religious or cultural background, the myth of Santa Claus is rooted in assumptions of how the world works. The myth goes something like this: "If you are a good child, you are going to be rewarded and receive a gift." In this case, the reward is a baby. The assumption that good things happen to good people may, in fact, push us to live morally upright lives, but it will not help us achieve pregnancy. One patient wept when she told me about her ne'er-do-well cousin:

> She has a history of drug abuse, dropped out of college, and can't seem to keep a job. How is it that she unintentionally gets pregnant and I—who have a master's degree, a spouse, and a career—cannot? This is entirely unfair!

If one thinks about the converse of the Santa myth—in other words, if you are not rewarded—does that mean that you are bad or have done something wrong? Most likely not, but so many people who have struggled with infertility or had a pregnancy loss find themselves questioning their past. "What did I do to deserve this?" is a question I have heard from many clients. In my therapy practice, rather than reassure someone that they likely did nothing wrong, I listen closely to the accounts of what they think they are being punished for. Self-blame can be staggering, but it can paradoxically feel better in explaining a pregnancy demise than having no viable reason for the loss at all.

Sometimes, people blame their current reproductive trauma on something that has happened in their past. You may question if perceived past indiscretions are the cause of your current loss. Some worry that they partied too much when they were younger; others worry that they were too promiscuous. If you have experienced previous trauma, that may also trigger self-blame. Marian, for example, was only a child when her parents divorced.

> I remember hearing my parents talk about money a lot. I always had the feeling that it was because of me that they didn't have enough money; that it was costing them too much—like for day care—because of me. In my 4-year-old mind, I thought I caused their divorce. I realize now—as an adult—that getting a divorce would not solve their financial problems, but it would actually increase them. But I always thought it was my fault.

Marian grew up blaming herself for the divorce. Taking responsibility for any negative events that occurred in her life became habitual. "I know that as a 4-year-old I wasn't at fault. I can see this pattern," she thoughtfully went on, "but I can't seem to stop myself from having these thoughts." It made sense that she would equate the stillbirth she experienced with these deeply entrenched beliefs. She felt responsible for destroying her family back then—the stillbirth triggered that sense of being at fault again.

Another issue that can set off self-blame is past sexual abuse. Nora, 36, and her wife, Pat, 42, sought out the care of a female reproductive specialist when they decided to start a family. The decision of who would carry the pregnancy was easy for them, both because of Nora's age and because Pat did not want to be pregnant. They chose a donor from a reputable sperm bank, hoping that Nora would become pregnant through intrauterine insemination (IUI). Nora said,

> I was nervous before the procedure—I think that's normal. What I didn't expect was to be flooded with a flashback from 20 years ago. I started to panic, thinking back to the rape when I was 16. I sat bolt upright on the exam table. Pat and our doctor were both taken off guard when I told them I had to leave.

Being sensitive to Nora's distress, they talked about postponing the procedure. Because everything was ready to go and Nora's cycle was at the perfect time, they went ahead with the IUI. Eight weeks later, Nora miscarried and was in the throes of self-blame when she came in for therapy. "For one thing, I was so stressed out during the IUI, how could it possibly have worked? Perhaps I don't deserve to be a mother. Here's proof that I can't protect my child. My womb is contaminated!" she cried. As we explored her past trauma and the self-blame associated with the rape, it became clear that the current stressors of getting pregnant followed by having a loss were overwhelming her. Her negative thinking about herself—that she did not deserve anything positive—was a challenging distortion that needed to be addressed.

Women who have had an abortion may also be at increased risk for self-blame. For example, Charlotte found herself in a very difficult position. She was getting ready to leave for college when she realized she was pregnant by her high school boyfriend. She felt so much shame.

> I knew better. It was a total mistake. Just one time we got carried away, and there I was with an unwanted pregnancy. I was so not ready to even consider being a parent; my sights were set on going to college. My boyfriend and I had even talked about breaking up, as we were going to different schools.

Her reproductive story at that time did not include having a baby as a teenager. Fast forward 15 years: Charlotte and her husband (not her former boyfriend) experienced a stillbirth. "Now that I'm ready to become a parent, my baby died. Did it have anything to do with the abortion?" she wondered.

The research on abortion has found that in most cases it does not increase risks to a woman's mental health, nor does it contribute to fertility problems or pregnancy complications (National Academies of Sciences, Engineering, and Medicine Committee on Reproductive Health Services, 2018). In fact, the overriding emotion based on women who receive an abortion is relief. The Turnaway Study was conducted with nearly 1,000 women who were seeking an abortion (Miller et al., 2020; Rocca et al., 2020). Some were able to get one, whereas others (who were over the gestational age limit) were not. Five years later, the women who wanted an abortion but couldn't access care struggled psychologically and financially. The Turnaway Study researchers found that significant long-term social and psychological trauma can occur when abortion is restricted (Miller et al., 2020; Rocca et al., 2020).

While Charlotte's abortion had nothing to do with her subsequent loss, she couldn't help but reflect on it:

> I know the abortion had been absolutely the right thing to do. I have no regrets about it. But I wonder if that was my only

> chance at becoming a mom. What if I had a baby when I was 18? My life would have been so different than it is now.

Feelings about previous abortions are often activated when faced with a current reproductive loss. Here again the reproductive story has taken a turn in an undesired direction. It is important to address these feelings, bring them to light, and process them.

If you have seen yourself in any of these vignettes, you are not alone. For all of us, our past influences the present—for better or worse—and impacts our reproductive stories. Imagining that you have done something to cause a pregnancy loss is emotionally unsettling and naturally causes a great deal of emotional pain. You need to know that it is highly unlikely that your past is related to your current reproductive loss. When I see people in therapy who think they deserve this trauma, I want to know more: What happened to them? Why do they feel they are being punished? Exploring these thoughts and feelings can foster healing—both of past trauma and the current one. In addressing negative emotions about oneself, we can work toward writing not just a new reproductive story but also a new narrative about one's life.

Core Belief 6: This Was Supposed to Be Easy

The assumption that pregnancy is the most natural thing in the world, and that everyone can do it if they want to, really sums up the fundamental beliefs about pregnancy. Discontinue using birth control, throw away the junk food, stop drinking alcohol, exercise but don't overdo it—that's what most of us believe is the right formula for having a successful pregnancy and childbirth. How is it possible that someone who has done everything right winds up delivering a premature baby or loses a fallopian tube as she suffers from an ectopic pregnancy? Why do some people seem to sail through this passage, while others face unanticipated storms and rough seas? Running into obstacles on the journey to parenthood was not the way it was supposed to be. This is not the way the story was supposed to go.

As mentioned previously, researchers in the field of trauma have compared the loss of basic assumptions—benevolence, predictability, and control—to an earthquake (Tedeschi & Calhoun, 2004). Using the earthquake metaphor, the foundations of these core beliefs can be reduced to rubble when a pregnancy loss occurs. Sadly, there seems to be no rhyme or reason for these losses. It can be hard to believe a doctor when they tell you it was just bad luck.

When earthquakes occur and cracks appear in what had been solid structures, and when windows break and shatter, we focus on the need to do repair work and rebuild. This takes considerable time and effort. Finding the right building materials to replace the roof, for example, is difficult no doubt, but finding the right materials to mend a broken heart is a very different task indeed. And it is anything but easy.

SUMMARY

When hopes and dreams about pregnancy are demolished, it can indeed feel like a shattered window that has been broken into tiny pieces. If you were able to put the pieces together again, it would certainly not look the same as it did originally. You may be able to see out of the window again, but you would also likely see the seams where the pieces were joined. The before piece of glass is different from the after reconstruction. People too have a sense of themselves before the trauma of pregnancy loss and after it. The trauma changes us, and not always for the worse, as we'll discuss in Chapter 8. As we heal, rebuild, and regain new meaning in our lives, there will still be scars present—just like the seams in the piece of glass. The scars may fade with time but will never be erased.

Learning about oneself and making sense of these losses is part of the rebuilding process. Old assumptions need to be revised to incorporate new realities; it may be difficult, but it is part of the healing that takes place. Recognizing pregnancy loss as a trauma can help you and the people around you understand how deeply you have been affected. It is not something that you can ignore or put behind you. These losses need to be grieved. In the next chapter, we'll explore how grieving a reproductive trauma and loss differs from grief in general. Not only are you grieving the loss of your child, but you are also mourning all that you had assumed—all the core beliefs that shaped your world before the loss—about pregnancy, childbirth, and parenting.

CHAPTER 4

HOW DO YOU GRIEVE YOUR BABY?

No one gets through life without experiencing some kind of loss. It may be the loss of a job, the loss of a relationship, or the loss of someone you love. These are painful and difficult emotional experiences that take time to heal from. Most of the losses people experience are that of our past—that is, the loss of people we have known and loved. The loss of a baby or a hoped-for baby, however, is different. It is the loss of the future. The loss of a baby goes against the natural cycle of life in which grandparents predecease parents and parents predecease children. There should have been a new little life cradled in your arms—a new beginning; but you have had to deal with death and demise—an ending that you never expected.

This is not the way you thought your story would unfold. It can feel as if your brain and your heart are on a continual play loop trying to understand the hows and whys of your loss. So many questions may be swirling through your head right now:

- How do I grieve a death when there should have been life?
- Why has this happened?
- What did I do to cause this?
- How do I grieve a baby who never was?
- What if I want to try again?

- How do I grieve when there are no rituals, or very few, to help guide me?
- How do I grieve when the people around me are at a loss for how to support me?

In this chapter, we'll try to answer these many questions. So little has been studied about how pregnancy losses differ from other deaths and hardships that occur. In part because of that, you may be ill-prepared for how to handle your feelings and those of others around you. Pregnancy loss is a unique experience that needs special attention (Cuenca, 2023). This chapter will help you learn how to put one foot in front of the other, how to create meaningful rituals for yourself and your family, and why there is an ache in your heart like no other. We'll focus first on grief in general; you will discover how theories and thoughts about grief have changed over time. We'll then address grief specific to your baby who has died, or to your hoped-for baby who was alive in your heart, and understand how to honor this deep connection that continues over time.

GRIEF AND ATTACHMENT

If there were some kind of scale that could measure love and loss, it would probably look something like Figure 4.1. Here, the upward rising line indicates the more love and attachment you feel for someone, the more grief and sadness you feel when they are gone. There is a direct relationship between how much you love someone and how much you hurt with their passing.

If only we could measure this vague notion of love. We all feel it, we all know it, but it may mean different things to each of us. It is not as if you can weigh it on a scale or calculate how much is in your bloodstream. And it may feel different depending on each relationship you have. The love you feel toward your parents may

FIGURE 4.1. Relationship Between Love and Intensity of Grief

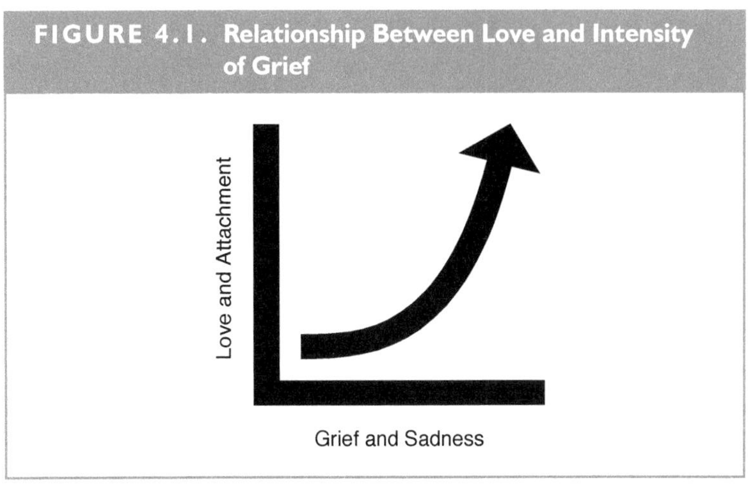

not feel the same as the love you feel toward your significant other, other members of your family, or your friends. This amorphous feeling present in all of us cannot truly be described, and yet it is a huge factor in what makes life meaningful and makes us human.

When you think about a loved one who has died, you may be filled with many memories—some may make you laugh or cry, some may make you angry, and some may fill you with regret. You can browse through photographs you have stored and realize that even though these loved ones are no longer with you, you will never forget them. It's the attachment you feel for your loved one that holds them dear to your heart.

In psychological terms, we call this *continuing bonds.* This means that we cannot—and we do not—completely disengage from the deceased. Mourners have a continued sense of connection with those who have died. You may even feel their presence at times—perhaps something occurs during the day that triggers a sense that they are with you. One person remarked that every time she saw a butterfly, it made her feel that her mother was there. You may find yourself talking about your loved one or even talking to them in your mind. You may seek their advice (e.g., How might your father have handled the situation at hand?) to help you weigh out decisions. These kinds of thoughts, feelings, or conversations are not abnormal; rather, they illustrate that a new relationship forms: In learning to live without the loved one, you can find comfort in their presence in your memories. Although their life has ended, your love for them goes on.

In the past, around the turn of the 20th century, Sigmund Freud (1912/2000) thought it best to sever the attachment to the deceased and work on building new relationships, almost as a replacement. Freud talked about the importance of *hypercathecting* (intensely expressing your feelings about the person) and then *decathecting* (detaching yourself emotionally from the person). Decathecting was thought to serve as a protective coping mechanism to avoid or lessen the pain of the loss, but later researchers who studied grief thought, "Is detachment really possible?" (Baker, 2001). Interestingly, although Freud wrote about these ideas in his work, in his own personal life, he admitted that the loss of a loved one would always leave a hole that could never find a substitute.

Post Freud, other concepts of grief took form, and his work was expanded on. For one thing, the notion that grief could be delayed or triggered by other current events in one's life became part of the understanding of how grief works. It was also understood that it is common for feelings to reemerge long after a death has occurred (Lindemann, 1944). The fact that grief knows no timeline is an important element when we consider continuing bonds. The acute grief you may experience after a loss may fade with time, but the feelings do not ever completely disappear—they may emerge after lying dormant and may be ongoing throughout your life.

Another researcher many of you may be aware of is Elisabeth Kübler-Ross. In her seminal work with people who had life-threatening diseases and were dying, she developed the idea that people go through different emotional stages at the end of their life (Kübler-Ross, 1969). The five stages she proposed are as follows:

1. Denial (This can't be happening to me.)
2. Anger (Why is this happening to me?)
3. Bargaining (If I promise to do better or take better care of myself, will I get well again?)
4. Despair or resignation (I understand that there is nothing I can do.)
5. Acceptance (I know I can't stop death from happening.)

According to Kübler-Ross, these stages follow one after the other, with each stage needing to be completed before moving on to the next. As illustrated in Figure 4.2, Kübler-Ross's model proposed that those at the end of their life move in a straight line from one stage to the next as they move closer to death.

It's important to remember that Kübler-Ross's (1969) model was meant to describe the grief experienced by the dying, not what was experienced by survivors. How is it different for those who are grieving the loss of a loved one? First, the stages do not necessarily occur in a set order. Also, not everyone experiences every stage, nor do they have to complete one stage before entering the next. As we can see in Figure 4.3, emotions may bounce back and forth, sometimes within the same day or even the same hour. This is perfectly normal. These feelings can be likened to a pinball machine: The lever is pulled and the feelings spring from one spot to another, triggering a leap to another emotion and back again. The greater the attachment to the loved one who has died, the more bells and whistles the pinball creates.

FIGURE 4.2. Stages of Grief for People at the End of Life

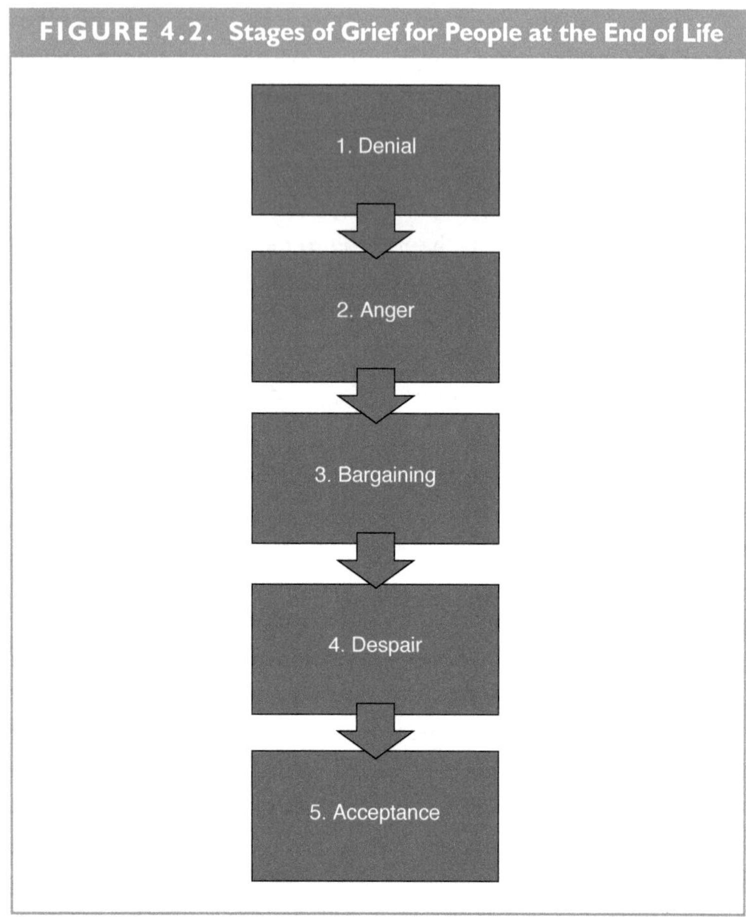

This "pinball brain," as I sometimes refer to it, happens to those who have experienced reproductive trauma. Patients have told me they feel like they are "going crazy," describing their emotions as being "all over the map." I reassure you—as I have countless patients—that no, you are not going crazy; this is a normal process that takes place when you have been traumatized by pregnancy loss.

FIGURE 4.3. Stages of Grief for Reproductive Losses

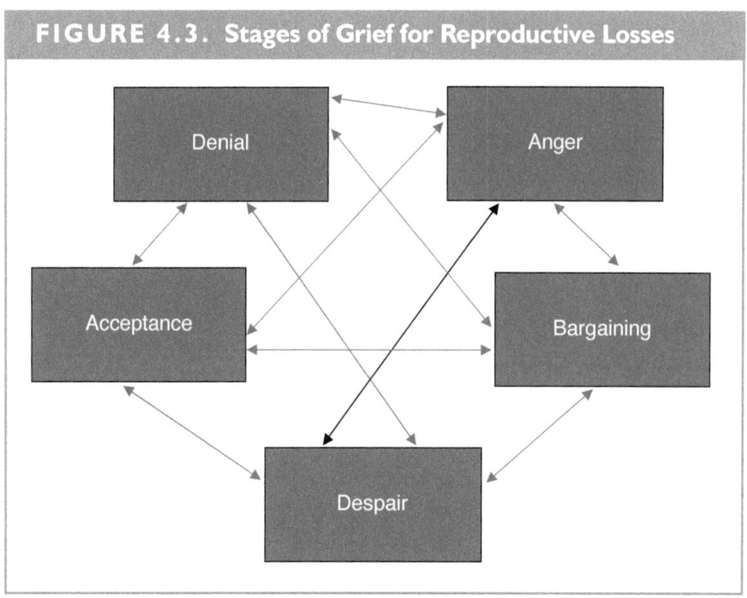

STAGES OF GRIEF AND PREGNANCY LOSS

Even though the stage model of grief does not happen sequentially with pregnancy loss, it can be helpful to look at each stage separately to understand what you are going through emotionally. We'll go through them in the same order as the Kübler-Ross (1969) model, but remember that these feelings may be happening simultaneously and repeatedly.

Denial

When a pregnancy loss occurs, the first reaction is often shock. Physically, you may experience weakness or dizziness or feel like you might faint. You might feel disengaged or removed from the news.

You may not be able to understand or process what you are being told. Some women have said the only thing they can remember hearing is that their baby no longer had a heartbeat—then they heard nothing else that was said. "I knew the doctor and my husband were having a conversation, but I didn't understand what they were talking about," said Meg. "It felt like I was underwater. I could hear sounds but not make sense of them."

Denial, which can serve as a protective mechanism, helping us through very tough situations, often goes along with shock. Denial is the feeling of disbelief; your loss just doesn't seem real. Meg went on to describe it:

> I knew it was not good news, but if I didn't allow the information in, maybe it would go away. Looking back on it, I wanted to believe that I was still pregnant, that I was still going to have a baby.

Denial is that feeling that the loss isn't actually occurring. On one level, you know the truth of the reality; on another, you may detach from it. It is just too overwhelming to bear. "This shouldn't be happening to me," Meg sobbed, "I took such good care of myself."

Trying to make sense out of the loss is part of grieving it. As Kübler-Ross (1969) suggested, denial is often the first stage of grief; however, even after time has passed and the reality of the loss has set in, there may be moments of returning to disbelief and shock.

Anger

What do you think about when you imagine someone who is grieving? How would you describe them? If you answered by saying a person would be tearful and sad, you would be correct. But other feelings also occur when grieving in general, and with a pregnancy loss specifically. Many people don't shed tears; in fact, what they do feel and outwardly express is anger. Take for example, Bill and his wife, Renee, who found out after their twin boys were born prematurely that they didn't survive. Bill had been so thrilled with the pregnancy but within days of the birth and death of his sons, he took a crowbar and sledgehammer and started demolishing a bathroom in their house. Although this had been on the list of home repairs he and his wife had wanted to do, the timing of it was totally out of line with what Renee expected and how she was feeling. It took some time for her to understand that this—the demolition and his anger—was an expression of his grief. Bill explained:

> I felt so helpless. I needed to bang, thrash, and destroy something because my boys were gone. I needed to feel like I could take some action and build something new. It's not like I thought this all out beforehand, but I needed to let off steam.

Even if anger isn't expressed in a physical way, like Bill did, feelings of resentment, irritation, and rage are normal and to be expected in grieving a reproductive loss. Maybe you are angry that your younger sister had a baby before you, when you had always done everything first in the family. Maybe you are furious that a friend, who knows you have been struggling to conceive, announced her pregnancy on social media and didn't talk to you privately about it. You may feel you have to distance yourself from a friend who complains all the time about her kids: Doesn't she get how much that hurts you? Perhaps you are angry because your parents didn't remember to call on the anniversary of when your baby died.

Sometimes the anger is free-floating, looking anywhere and everywhere to latch on. Situations like someone cutting you off on the road now may fill you with rage, where in the past you might have just muttered under your breath. Or maybe you blow up at a coworker because she leaves a mess in the break room every day. Sometimes the anger gets turned inward. When this happens, there is a tendency to blame oneself for the loss. Anger turned against oneself may manifest with depression and helplessness. As discussed in Chapter 3, finding fault with oneself can oddly feel more comforting than not having any reason for the loss. "I am just angry with the world," wailed Sophie. "This is so unfair!" Sophie's cry can be echoed over and over by people who experience pregnancy loss.

Bargaining

Listening to Sophie's story, it makes sense why she was so angry. At 42 years old, she needed to terminate her pregnancy because of early-onset preeclampsia. This was a much-wanted pregnancy; after trying on their own, she and her partner turned to in vitro fertilization to achieve it. On a routine prenatal visit, her doctor noted that her blood pressure was elevated. Urine tests indicated excess protein. When Sophie complained of having severe headaches, some blurry vision, and pain in her belly, her doctor was alarmed and explained the risks involved in continuing the pregnancy. As gently as she could, Sophie's doctor said,

> This is not good news. You may not be able to take it all in right now, but I'm very concerned about you and your baby. If you were close to the end of your pregnancy, it would be one thing, and I would schedule delivery for right now. But because you are in the middle of your pregnancy, we need to consider termination of it for your health. Early-onset preeclampsia is very serious and can be life-threatening if you don't terminate.

After Sophie recovered from the procedure, her health returned to normal. While physically she felt fine, her grief was overwhelming. As noted, she was very angry and upset. She also wondered if her decision to terminate was really necessary. She kept asking herself what-if questions: "What if I had known about my blood pressure earlier? Would that have made a difference?" "What about my diet?" "Work was so stressful. What if I had quit?" "If only we had tried getting pregnant when I was younger." These are the types of questions and self-reflections that people do in the bargaining stage. People also find themselves making deals with themselves. For example, Sophie decided that if she were able to get pregnant again, she would stop working immediately. This was her attempt to assert some control over the situation. In truth, her work stressors likely did not impact the pregnancy in any way, but this is an example of how one bargains in grief: "If I do it differently, if I do it better, if I am a better person—then maybe the outcome will be different."

Despair

The despair phase of grief can be described as feelings of hopelessness and helplessness. With sadness, you may feel that there is nothing you can do to change the situation or fix it. Despair may make you not care about anything and feel as if the future holds no hope. It is true that the feelings around reproductive traumas and losses can become global—in other words, it can be difficult to differentiate the specific sadness around your loss from a universal darkness of bereavement. The risk of clinical depression following a pregnancy loss or other reproductive trauma is high. For those who have had a stillbirth, 50% experience depression and anxiety in the first few months following the loss, and they may continue feeling the effects 3 years later (Hughes et al., 2002). Another study compared those who had a stillbirth or neonatal death with a control group of women with live births (Gold et al., 2016). Not surprisingly, the rate of depression was four times higher, and the rate of posttraumatic stress was seven times higher, in women who had a loss (Gold et al.,

2016). Yet another study surveyed men and women at fertility clinics, and researchers found that more than half of women and nearly a third of men were suffering from depression (Pasch et al., 2016).

It is difficult to hold out hope when your dreams have been crushed, when your reproductive story has come up against barriers, defeat, and death. Adding to these negative feelings, you may feel alone in it all. As we'll discuss in the next chapter, even if you and your spouse or partner have both been dealt the same blow, you may crawl into your own corners and not share it with each other. Just as the two of you have your own unique reproductive stories, you have your own coping mechanisms and ways to express grief. If you and your partner are not on the same page, it can lead to even more feelings of despair.

What is crucial to remember is that this stage of grief is not permanent. There are ways to move forward, ways to heal from these losses. As will be discussed in this book, there are many opportunities to edit and rewrite your reproductive story, whether that includes a child in your future or not. It is often out of the depths of despair that new possibilities emerge, ones that you may not have realized were available to you before.

Acceptance

The acceptance stage is about acknowledging the fact that your life has changed. Acceptance is often considered the final stage of grief. It is marked by the knowledge that you can't change what has happened, but you can make decisions about your new reality. With the passing of time, it is only natural to try to figure out what comes next. While it may become easier to live with the loss over time, remember that grief doesn't ever really end and it is not linear.

So often, you may think you're doing okay, carrying on, and even planning for the future, but then something triggers you and the intensity of feelings of loss return. Perhaps a stranger asks if you have children, or your mother calls and says, "You'll never guess who's pregnant!" You may find yourself more upset when an anniversary of the loss rolls around or during holidays. Situations like these can feel like a setback, but they are normal and to be expected. In fact, if you can anticipate vulnerable times, you may be able to manage them better. Exercise 4.1 offers some suggestions on how to get through hypothetical challenging events.

EXERCISE 4.1. Letting Others Know What You Need

Imagine you are approaching what would have been your due date. That is often such a difficult time, especially the first time that date rolls around. It can be hard not to imagine how your life would be different if your pregnancy had gone to full term with a healthy baby at the end. While your due date may be emblazoned in your mind, others may not keep track of it. What would make you feel that this date is acknowledged? What would make you feel cared for? What do you think would be the best strategy for ensuring that your needs get met? Is it possible to ask for what you want? If you have expectations of others that don't get met, it can make matters worse. If you are concerned, for example, that those close to you will not remember the date, perhaps you can gently remind them and let them know how painful it is for you. Maybe you initiate a hike with a friend or carve out time for coffee with your partner. What makes sense for you?

Another triggering time is the anniversary of your pregnancy demise or the baby's death. As will be discussed in the next sections, how you mark these moments is also significant. Whether you do so in private or have others participate is up to you. Again, the first step is to identify what makes sense to you. Developing rituals to honor your pregnancy and baby that are comforting to you does not necessarily take the pain away, but they are a way of recognizing all that has happened. With each subsequent year, rituals allow you to build new memories and note how life has gone on.

COMMEMORATING THE DEAD

Every culture and religion has ways to honor and celebrate the lives of loved ones who have died. For some, rituals are believed to help the deceased move on to the next life, while other traditions are focused on helping and supporting the bereaved. These practices often bring people together not only to share in the grief but also to reflect on the deceased's life. As difficult as it is to lose a loved one, we have memories to hold on to. Rituals help the bereaved to focus and reflect on those memories. At funerals and memorials, for example, an oral eulogy is often given; stories are told about the person's life, their accomplishments, and their character. Like pearls on a necklace, the stories build on each other and connect us to the person we loved—and continue to love. There may be written accounts of a person's life as well. An obituary is an article typically written by family or friends, often published in a newspaper or online, which highlights the person's life. This process is not easy and many tears will be shed, but these established rites help people through difficult times. Unfortunately, there are few, if any, rituals in place for pregnancy loss.

WHEN A BABY OR HOPED-FOR BABY DIES

When a baby dies or a pregnancy fails, what are the memories we hold? Often, they are just painful and frightening. There is no recounting of a person's life and character; rather, you may be haunted by sights, sounds, smells, and experiences that are anything but upbeat. You may not be able to shake the image of blood in the toilet or the stunned look on a sonographer's face. Memories may consist of being rushed into a hospital emergency room for a delivery without hearing a baby's cry at the end of it all. None of these are positive, none are pleasant.

Another difference is that rather than causing people to come together, pregnancy losses are often experienced alone. Sometimes the only people who know what is happening are the woman, her partner if there is one, and perhaps her doctor. When I pause to think about this, it is so startling. Here is someone experiencing one of the most life-shattering events possible, and no one knows. Consider, for example, a woman who is having an early miscarriage. Externally, she seems the same as always, but from the inside, her entire world has turned upside down. She has experienced a profound, yet private, loss. There is nothing to eulogize, and there is no obituary to write. Just as there are few if any memories, there are virtually no rituals to guide her through grief.

Just as startling is how pregnancy loss was dealt with in the past. Prior to the 1970s, grief following a miscarriage or stillbirth was often just not acknowledged. These life-altering incidents were treated as nonevents: Stillborn babies, for example, were routinely whisked out of sight. The intention—which was supported by family, friends, and even the medical community—was to spare parents from the distress of seeing their baby. Parents were told to get on with their lives, especially in the case of miscarriage (Brownlee & Oikonen, 2004). Pay no mind to all those feelings! They were told it was best to push down their emotions, truly an impossible task. In reality, it left those who had experienced pregnancy loss feeling confused and unsupported. Indeed, it silenced people from acknowledging the obvious: A devastating loss just occurred.

Imagine what it was like for those who were coping with infertility. If patients described stillbirth or miscarriage as shrouded in silence, then infertility struggles were experienced in a void or vacuum. People spoke in hushed tones about couples who didn't have children. Adoption was the only option available at that time. I can remember when I was a child hearing adults say things like, "They had to adopt" or "Those kids are adopted." It was said in such a way that

I looked askance at those kids, as if something was wrong with them. It is painful to think back on it now. Did those children feel less than? What about their parents? The societal shame surrounding fertility issues still exists today but was much worse in the past.

GRIEVING A STILLBIRTH OR DEATH OF A NEWBORN VERSUS AN EARLY PREGNANCY LOSS OR INFERTILITY

This section examines the similarities and differences between grieving a stillbirth and the death of an infant versus grieving a miscarriage and infertility. Although feelings overlap in all these situations, divergences in ways of mourning occur when there is no body to grieve over.

Grieving a Stillbirth or Newborn Death

Gone are the days when parents' grief was pushed aside and minimized. Nowadays, there is more and more understanding of just how crushing these events are. Pregnancy loss is now recognized as a significant trauma. There is a growing awareness of the depth of attachment that occurs long before a baby's birth. Think back to the origins of your own reproductive story; the bond between you and your baby-to-be may have existed prior to conception, prior even to a committed relationship. It is a connection so deep, it is a part of your identity. This strong link between your baby and your sense of self may not be fully recognized until the bond is broken with a reproductive loss.

Because of the growing understanding of the impact of stillbirth and the death of a newborn baby on parents, hospital procedures have changed. Rather than whisking a baby away, these days it is common practice for hospital staff, nurses, and midwives to encourage parents to see and hold their stillborn baby or premature baby who has died. You may have been hesitant to do so, but most people report that even if they are initially reluctant, they appreciate having this opportunity. It is one of the ways your baby and this experience can feel real. In fact, you would not be alone if you felt you didn't have enough time with your baby. Research suggests that parents have fewer symptoms of anxiety and depression if they can spend time with their baby (Kingdon et al., 2015). Sometimes, due to medical complications, parents are not able to see or hold their child; these parents can feel as if they were robbed of the time to connect with their infant.

Another recommended practice is to take photographs of your child. Although this too may feel strange at first, it is another way to validate your baby's existence. Many parents take pictures with their phones, but there are also professional photographers who offer this service. One couple described their experience of having a photographer in the room with them:

> We were so overwhelmed and in shock when our baby was stillborn. Did we really want a stranger in the room with us? But they were so discrete that at a certain point we forgot they were even there. And now we have the most amazing pictures of our beautiful little girl.

Another way to memorialize your baby is to create a memory box. Many hospitals help do this by taking prints or casts of your baby's hands, feet, or both. You can also include a hospital bracelet, some clothing, a lock of hair, or photographs. You might want to include a poem or a letter to your baby. Sometimes people will continue to add to their box each year—perhaps writing another letter on each anniversary date. These physical remembrances can provide some solace. It can help make this trauma into something tangible that you can revisit at any time.

The mourning process for a stillbirth or a newborn loss is facilitated by the reality of the baby's body. You may choose to have a funeral service in your place of worship, or you may decide to create your own memorial service. Having people around you who love and care about you is so important. Whether there is a formal service or something else you create, those feelings of love can grow as you share this time with people close to you. One couple had a small gathering at the beach. Each person there wrote a personal message to the baby, then the couple placed her ashes, along with the messages, in a cannister and sent her spirit out to sea. Another family, on the anniversary date of their baby's death, visited the gravesite and brought flowers, sat for a while, and reflected on how life had changed because of their experience. Yet another family planted a flowering bush that blooms each year during the anniversary of their baby's birth and death.

Perhaps you create a tradition of opening and adding to your baby's memory box each year. Whatever you decide on—whether you have a formal funeral or create your own memorial—it needs to be meaningful for you. Sometimes families decide to have a funeral in addition to establishing a ritual of their own creation. Whatever you have chosen to do, these rituals are ways to honor your child and bring people together to support you and each other. They validate your loss. They also can create new memories: With each passing year, you can think back on your experience and the continuation of your feelings and bond with your baby.

Grieving an Early Pregnancy Loss or Infertility

If you have had a miscarriage, an ectopic pregnancy, or other early-term pregnancy loss, your feelings may be just as intense as someone who has suffered a late-term loss. Likewise, if you have struggled with infertility, the pain you feel can be devastating with each passing cycle and each passing month. As we talk more about these types of losses, you will see that although the feelings are not less intense, one big difference is that they are less recognized as traumatic events by society at large. These losses tend to be less openly talked about—in large part because women feel enormous shame, as if they were at fault for causing the pregnancy demise. We know that most miscarriages, for example, are caused by a genetic or chromosomal anomaly and not by anything a woman did or did not do. Yet self-blame and shame are such common reactions when these losses occur. As one patient described it,

> I had no idea how many women have had miscarriages until I had one. Whenever I mention it, someone always tells me about their own story. Why didn't I know about this "club" before? It's almost like a secret society where you have to know the password to enter. Why don't women talk about it?

These losses fall under what mental health professionals call *disenfranchised grief* (Doka, 1989). Disenfranchised grief is any type of grief that is not publicly recognized or acknowledged. An example could be someone who is divorced and experiencing grief if their former spouse passes away. Feelings exist but may not be understood by others. Anyone who has experienced infertility or early pregnancy loss is at risk for disenfranchised grief. As mentioned earlier, it may be that no one even knows that you were trying to conceive or had been pregnant. These losses, although not less meaningful, are less tangible. As agonizing as a stillbirth or the death of an infant is to parents, the mourning process is facilitated by the reality of the baby's body. When there is no actual body to mourn over, grief can feel illegitimate. This can become even more difficult if you have been told by well-meaning people, including medical personnel, to move on or not to dwell on it, or if they offer other advice that negates your feelings of loss. This advice is meant to make you feel better, although it does not. In their own way, people are trying to fix it and make it better for you. In the absence of rules for this kind of loss, they may not know how to manage it either and find themselves stumbling in their effort to help. What people who haven't experienced this kind of loss often do not understand is that it isn't something you can just shut out of your mind, as if it will magically disappear.

"Am I even allowed to grieve?" asked Akiko, who miscarried twice, once at 6 weeks and then again several months later at 8 weeks. "With the first miscarriage, I thought 'Okay—just bad luck.' These things happen. But when it happened again, I was floored. What is going on? What did I do wrong?" she asked. It was 6 months after the second miscarriage when Akiko started therapy with me. It had been a miserable time for her. She isolated a lot, finding hosts of reasons not to see friends. "I just wasn't up for it. They didn't know—because I didn't tell them—what we've been going through. It's private—and embarrassing. And I don't want anyone's advice." I reassured her:

> I'm not here to give you advice, but to let you know that your grief is real. And to let you know that there is no easy way to get through this. There's no magic wand I can wave to make it all better—believe me, I wish there were. But I do know that the more you can understand why you are hurting, the more you can see that your dreams have been blown up, the more you'll be able to heal. Allowing yourself to talk about it and to grieve is a big part of this.

Grieving early pregnancy losses and the losses surrounding infertility can be more complicated than grieving stillbirth or infant death—there are no funerals, no sitting shiva, no sanctioned ways of joining with others in grief. There are virtually no religious or cultural rituals to follow. Although you may have looked to others for how they processed these kinds of losses, you may not even want to admit that you've had a loss. As Akiko mentioned, she was embarrassed to let others know, as if having a miscarriage was a reflection on her. Holding these feelings in and avoiding others can lead to increased depression and anxiety. On the other hand, talking about these losses—with someone you trust—is a way to destigmatize them. These losses are statistically so common and yet so misunderstood. Sharing your experience with others can help ease the burden.

Aside from talking about the trauma, it is possible to create rituals for yourself—and if you want to, include your loved ones—to validate your loss. When I work with individuals or couples in trying to create a ritual, the most important thing is that it be meaningful to them. What works for someone else may not be right for you. Akiko, for example, needed to find something that she could do by herself. She didn't even want to involve her partner—at least in the beginning. We explored what she thought might be helpful based on things she had done in the past. What were some things she loved to do that brought her peace and feelings of accomplishment? "I guess one thing that always seems to help is working in the garden," she reflected. "I find it cathartic to pull weeds, believe it or not." We talked more about her garden and what she liked to grow, and I asked Akiko what pulling weeds might symbolize to her. "What do you mean?" she asked. "Pulling weeds gives everything else a better chance to grow."

I agreed and added, "Pulling weeds also brings order to gardens. It's one of the things that makes them beautiful. Not only do you help plants grow, but you also get to control what you want to nurture." She paused and applied the metaphor to her own grief. "I get it. You are so right. It really does feel like my life has been out of control. Getting rid of the weeds in my head, in my heart, so to speak—maybe that's a start." Taking care of her garden with a new intention then became a daily ritual for Akiko.

CREATING A RITUAL FOR YOURSELF

How do you find a way to grieve that makes sense for you? If you can have a traditional burial, does that feel like enough? And if there are no sanctioned ways to mourn, as in the case of early pregnancy loss and infertility, how do you find something meaningful?

As with Akiko, the first step is reflecting on how you have managed stressful situations in the past. What has helped you cope? Do you prefer to manage on your own, or is it helpful for you to be with other people? Who are the people in your life that you can turn to? Who do you trust? Perhaps you need both solitude and the company of others; knowing yourself and respecting your needs is key to working through grief.

Once you have identified what you need, finding a way to translate that into some kind of personal ritual is the next step. As with Akiko and gardening, it may be something that you already do on a regular basis, but with focus on the activity with new intent. For others, creating a new tradition specifically related to their pregnancy loss helps with the mourning process.

Here are some things that people have created to commemorate their pregnancy loss. These are just ideas. What is critical is that the ritual makes sense to you.

- Celeste and Rick made a pact to go out to dinner each month, when she got her period. This was in no way a celebratory evening, but it was a way for them to acknowledge the issue. It created a time and place for them to support each other and keep communication open. As we will discuss in Chapter 5, couples can be at odds with each other when a loss occurs, whether it is because of infertility or other reproductive trauma. Connecting with each other in this monthly ritual was a positive way for Celeste and Rick to foster their relationship.

- Phil and Christopher decided to join a community garden in honor of the miscarriage their surrogate had. They said, "It felt good to watch something grow surrounded by other people at work in the garden. It gives us a moment of solace each time we go."
- "We decided to honor our little angel by donating toys to kids in the hospital," said Sam. "We've been doing it once a year ever since our first daughter, Bridgette, was stillborn. We suggested that our family—siblings and parents—do it as well. We all still give even though we were eventually able to have other children. Bridgette lives on through these donations."
- Rosa said, "I started to keep a journal after my ectopic pregnancy. It has given me a place to write about all my feelings—the good and the bad."
- After having three miscarriages within 2 years, Marjorie felt shaken and alone. She said, "I started therapy to help cope with these losses. It has now become a ritual—every Thursday at 3:00 p.m., without fail, I see my therapist. I get to tell my story over and over, and I am learning how these losses have affected my entire outlook on life."

SUMMARY

Pregnancy loss can take us by surprise. People don't usually anticipate that this will be a factor in their reproductive story. As we've discussed, the very foundations of what you believe—about pregnancy, about your life, about what is important—can feel like they are tottering and slipping away. To rebuild and restructure your life after a pregnancy loss, you need to grieve.

Grieving a reproductive loss is not simple, and it is so different from grieving other types of losses. This is true, in part, because there are few, if any, sanctioned ways to grieve pregnancy loss. It is so often wrapped up in silence, but it is important to know that you did not cause the loss. You are not at fault. Bottled up with disgrace, you may feel as if you need permission to grieve. The more you can release your feelings, however scary that might be, the more the shame around your loss can be lessened.

There may be concerns that as your life moves forward, you will forget about this loss. While you might go on to have other children, the attachment you feel toward the baby who has died or the hoped-for baby in your heart will always be there. Continuing that bond, understanding how important that child has been to you, will help you appreciate the rest of what life has in store.

As discussed throughout this chapter, grieving reproductive losses can be complex and filled with uncertainty, self-blame, and isolation. Added to this, couples, who have experienced the same loss, may have very different ways of managing and expressing their grief. In Chapter 5, we'll focus on how men and women may process these losses differently and how all couples can find common ground when misunderstandings arise.

CHAPTER 5

WE ARE NOT ON THE SAME PAGE: WHEN COUPLES GRIEVE REPRODUCTIVE LOSSES DIFFERENTLY

Even though you and your partner share a reproductive loss, you may manage and cope with it in vastly different ways. The very person you usually turn to in times of distress—your partner—may not be emotionally available, bringing you even more pain and isolation. This happens all the time, in both heterosexual and same-sex couples, and it doesn't necessarily mean that there is something inherently wrong with your relationship. It just means that you are both grieving in different ways from each other. Because there is no one right way to grieve, it can be confusing and lead to misunderstandings when one person is grieving one way and the other is grieving in a completely different way. In this chapter, we explore ways to increase empathy for your partner, better understand each other, and learn effective means of communication. We'll also focus on intimacy—sexual and otherwise—and how to mend connections with your partner when bonds feel shaky.

MEN AND WOMEN: STEREOTYPES AND GRIEF

Tearful, sorrowful, depressed, heartbroken—these are some of the ways we talk about a grief-stricken person.[1] They describe the classic image of someone who is grieving. Sitting with head in hands, staring off into space, wanting to isolate—in this state of mind, it is difficult to function and do much of anything. We know, however, that there are many other ways that people express their grief: They may get angry and irritated, or they may feel resentful and helpless. They may fight off their despair by taking action and getting things done. How can these seemingly diametrically opposed reactions both fall under the rubric of grief?

Researchers initially categorized these responses into masculine and feminine models of grief (Rando, 1985, 1986). On the surface, there do seem to be gender differences in how people grieve; but as we take a deeper dive into the theoretical models of grief and gender in this chapter, you'll see how the stereotypical understanding of men and women's grief has changed. Why is this important for you to know? The hope is it will help you understand what your partner is going through, and with a better understanding comes a better relationship.

Masculine–Feminine Model of Grief

When I imagine the masculine model of grief (Rando, 1985, 1986), I immediately think about John Wayne—the tough guy who through great bravery and gallantry overcomes criminals in his effort to do

---

[1]A note about language: In this section, I refer to *men* and *women* for simplicity and, in part, because much of the research I cite has been done on cisgender men and women. It is understood, however, that gender is a continuum and that not all individuals will fall into these categories. It is also understood that not all people who can become pregnant identify as women.

good. Or maybe you envision characters like Luke Skywalker or Harry Potter who strive to ward off evil and save the world. These heroes meet the enemy head on and make sacrifices, but they never give up. If the enemy here is the loss of a pregnancy, men's reactions may be described as striving to keep a stiff upper lip. Men who have experienced a reproductive loss are typecast as the stoic partner, the one who is strong for their grieving spouse. Their job is to support their wife or partner. If, for example, a funeral needs to be planned, men would be the ones to make the arrangements, call the family, and take care of any necessary plans. The research points to men's need to avoid emotional displays; men process their reactions through thought, not feeling (Rando, 1985, 1986). One of the problems with classifying men's grief this way is that their experience of loss can be readily overlooked. Is it that men are truly not emotional, or is it that societal rules presume their feelings are minimal? "I was expected to support her," said Greg after he and his wife experienced a stillbirth, "and I am happy to do so. Of course, I am there for her. But people ask me all the time how she's doing. What about me? I've got feelings too, you know." The perception that men only serve a supportive role is prevalent but unjustified. Research has shown that men may also blame themselves and feel the need to hide their feelings of sadness and distress (McCreight, 2004).

So much of the focus is on the woman's experience of pregnancy loss. After all, she is the one who has gone through the physical trials of the pregnancy. Her body has been put through so much—whether the loss happens with a hospital delivery or a miscarriage at home. Even for couples going through infertility treatments, women's bodies bear the lion's share of the interventions, and women receive ongoing reminders of treatment not working when their monthly menses occurs. The feminine model of grief puts feelings front and center (Rando, 1985, 1986). Women are expected to shed tears and want to process their emotions. The characteristics that we readily associate with grief—sadness, depressed mood, helplessness—classify the feminine model (Rando, 1985, 1986). If the masculine model can be illustrated by the hero stereotype, then the feminine model looks more like the damsel-in-distress stereotype. She is the one who needs support and comfort. Although this may be true, it is also true that would-be fathers need the same kind of care.

Intuitive–Instrumental Model of Grief

Let's look at another model: the *intuitive–instrumental model of grief* (Doka & Martin, 2011). Although it is related to gender, it is not necessarily determined by it. Instead of comparing men and women, this model compares two different styles or reactions to grief. The *intuitive griever* has similar features to the feminine model. The characteristics here are marked by tearfulness, sadness, and depressed mood. The *instrumental griever* is like the masculine model just described—more focused on finding solutions and avoiding emotional displays. The intuitive–instrumental model suggests that both intuitive and instrumental styles are present in both men and women (Doka & Martin, 2011). This is not limited to heterosexual cisgender couples; the pattern can occur with same-sex couples as well.

Think of it as a kind of seesaw. A person's expression of each style may vary from moment to moment, moving from one side to the other—this happens to all of us. As with the stages of grief we discussed in Chapter 4, which can change from one moment to the next, you may experience both intuitive and instrumental aspects of grief. How you convey grief can depend on your prominent expressive style and the type of loss that has occurred. The point is that each of us experiences varying degrees of both intuitive and instrumental grief. Sometimes, you may be ready to take a step out into the world again; at other times, you may feel like you are deep in a forest with no path through the trees. You may feel ready to try getting pregnant again one day, but then be overwhelmed with fear the next.

This pattern happens within everyone, but it also occurs between couples. What I have witnessed time and again in working with couples is that they may literally take turns in how they feel, switching back and forth between the intuitive and instrumental styles. When one is up, the other is down and vice versa. When one says, "Let's go," the other says, "No way." Does this sound familiar? These contrasting feelings can reveal themselves over seemingly small decisions, but it's the big decisions that can be so troublesome. Knowing about this pattern may help you better understand how you are processing your own grief as well as supporting your partner through theirs.

WHEN COUPLES DON'T SEE EYE TO EYE

No matter what your relationship is like, you and your partner are not clones of each other. You each have your own reproductive story, your own way of seeing the world, your own way of coping with hardships, and your own ways of expressing grief. Although there are numerous mourning rituals, religious or otherwise, there is simply no one right way to grieve. One person's reaction to loss may look very different from another's. I want to stress this point: Just because your reaction is not the same as your partner's, it doesn't mean that they are not grieving as intensely as you. Their grief just appears different, and it may also change with time. Trying to process your own grief is challenging enough. At the same time, making sense of your partner's feelings can seem like you are walking on eggshells, so to speak—unsure of every step you take.

SAME LOSS, DIFFERENT REACTIONS—OR ARE THEY?

The following vignettes highlight misunderstandings when couples are at odds with each other's grief reactions. Missteps and arguments happen all the time in relationships, especially when a reproductive trauma has occurred. The goal, of course, is to work through these painful moments and land on the same page again.

Renee and Bill: Emotional Wrestling Match

Let's think back to a couple we met in Chapter 4, Renee and Bill, who had premature twin boys who did not survive. Do you remember Bill's response? He took a sledgehammer to the bathroom; this horrified Renee, who was grieving in a more traditional way. What she needed was support—someone who would make her the proverbial cup of tea, someone who could be gentle and soothe her. In contrast, Bill felt like a trapped animal, and he needed to let out his rage. Renee's tears only intensified the explosion he was feeling inside. He needed to act and do something; she needed to retreat to a safe place to allow her wounds to heal. Neither of them openly verbalized their needs; rather, they assumed the other would know what would help.

Bill's anger was like dried kindling, spreading like wildfire and igniting fury in Renee. In a way, his anger forced her out of her tearful state by sparking her rage. She blew up at him: "What is wrong with you?" she screamed, "Are you out of your mind?" A blowup ensued, with each hurling out hurtful sentiments at each other and both yelling: "You are always so controlling! Everything has to be your way. You never think about me!" At a certain point, Bill broke down and sobbed: "I just can't believe this is happening!" A silence fell over the room then as the mood changed, and they both started to cry. At that moment, Bill's anger faded, and the more intuitive aspect of his grief emerged.

What just happened here? It started out with Renee and Bill in seemingly different corners, as if they were competing in an emotional wrestling match. Renee and Bill were reacting to the loss of their twins in their own ways, apart from each other and alone—on opposing sides of the ring. Bill's anger and rage began the fight. Observing this, it may seem that they were moving further away from each other. However, even though they were arguing, they were actually engaged with each other, perhaps for the first time since the trauma of their loss. Coming together, even though it was initially in anger, allowed them to connect in their grief. The connection deepened when they both started to cry.

Here is the takeaway from this example: Under feelings of anger, sadness exists; similarly, under feelings of sadness, anger is present. What seem like diametrically opposed emotions simmer in all of us—to different degrees at different times. For Renee and Bill, coming together like this allowed them to realize that they were not enemies of each other; rather, they were two people with shattered dreams who were trying their best to cope.

Ellie and Rob: The Need Not to Talk

Ellie and Rob had been struggling with infertility. They went through an in vitro fertilization (IVF) procedure, got pregnant, but then miscarried. Throughout their fertility journey, Rob's anxiety skyrocketed as he tried to support Ellie. He knew how difficult the IVF was, as a spectator to the shots and discomfort they caused. After the loss, he tried to comfort her but was struggling to know exactly how. Rob knew there were times that Ellie wanted to talk: He did his best to engage with her at those times, but there were just as many times when he needed not to talk. One of those moments is described next.

It was a scorchingly hot day. Rob had just walked in the door after a stressful day at work, followed by a harrowing commute with lots of traffic. He had been thinking about a cold beer all the way home. He wanted to relax, but when he opened the door to their apartment, he heard Ellie on the phone in tears. "That was your sister on the phone," Ellie said, coldly. "She was surprised because I didn't know about her pregnancy. How long have you known?" Rob felt like he'd been punched in the gut. "I'm so sorry. I was going to tell you but . . .," he muttered.

"But what!?" Ellie, now angry and sobbing, headed to the bedroom and shut the door. Rob's efforts to engage with Ellie fell flat; he felt angry as well because she was shutting him out. He knew she needed some time to cool off, as did he, but again he didn't know what to do. Feeling helpless and at a loss as to how to fix this mess, he got himself that beer and flopped down in front of the TV. How did Ellie react to Rob watching TV? To her, it was confirmation—albeit erroneous—that he just didn't care.

In this scenario, why do you think Rob did not tell Ellie about his sister's pregnancy? After all, he knew she was going to find out eventually. The truth is, he didn't want to upset her. Rob thought that not telling Ellie the news of his sister's pregnancy was a way for him to protect Ellie, at least in the short term. When Rob's sister told him she was pregnant, his heart sank. It wasn't just Ellie who needed to be shielded from this new reality; he needed it as well. This was one of those times when he needed not to talk—to shut down his own feelings as well as hide them from Ellie—but his avoidance and attempts at protection backfired.

How could Rob let Ellie know that a song had come on the radio on his commute to work that made him cry? If she knew how upset he was, wouldn't that make it worse for her? The need to keep a stiff upper lip and not let her know his true feelings—so culturally entrenched in men—was what he thought was expected of him. Research has been done on this phenomenon of keeping one's feelings under wraps so as not to upset the other; in psychological terms, this is known as *partner-oriented self-regulation* (POSR; Stroebe et al., 2013). Stroebe et al. looked specifically at bereaved parents and observed that one person in the relationship may suppress—or regulate—their own feelings to protect the other person. In other words, Rob worried that if Ellie knew the true extent of how sad he was, she would be even more upset; but in fact, just the opposite was true.

The multiple misunderstandings that can happen here are profound. Ellie interpreted Rob's silence about his sister's pregnancy to mean he felt it was unimportant. She wondered if that meant he not only didn't care about their loss but also didn't care about her. Did he even want to start a family anymore? This was far from the truth: Rob did want a family but didn't feel he could talk about it. The less Rob communicated, the more depressed Ellie felt. Researchers have found that not only does POSR increase their partner's grief, but it also increases a person's own grief (Stroebe et al., 2013). Suppressing negative feelings only seems to magnify them.

This vignette exemplifies how misinterpretations can be magnified. Although there may be times when the need not to talk should be respected, there are times when what seems like an effort to protect one's partner by not sharing can backfire. Of course, there will be moments when we just need to veg out, shutting out as much as we possibly can. We all need that from time to time. Psychologists and other mental health professionals tend to promote communication; the whole idea of talk therapy is to talk! Over the years, however, I have come to value silence and the need to recognize it not as a fault but rather as yet another way of coping. In this case, it was important for Ellie to have empathy for Rob; he was doing the best he could in his effort to protect her from more pain. Yet Rob needed to understand how his silence, especially about his sister's pregnancy, left Ellie feeling abandoned and alone.

As I discuss later in this chapter, I often suggest that couples try to begin conversations by asking, "Is this a good time to talk?"

If you try this and both of you are in accord, no problem. It is helpful, however, to have an agreement ahead of time that if one person is not emotionally available at that moment, then the discussion should be delayed. Picking a time to talk—and sticking to it—allows both of you to feel ready to tackle difficult situations and feelings.

Susan and Maggie: The Emotional Seesaw

Let's look at another couple to see the effects of POSR. Susan and her wife, Maggie, were thrilled when Maggie conceived on their first try using a donor they found through a sperm bank. Maggie described herself as a go-getter kind of person: Set your mind to something and you will succeed. "I've had to overcome many obstacles in my life," she said. "Being gay in a conservative family, I worked hard at making sure my family understood and supported me." Getting pregnant on her first try fit her ideas of how life should go, but losing that pregnancy at 10 weeks did not.

Maggie's negative feelings about herself were compounded by a disruption in her relationship with Susan. After the loss, Maggie took a leave of absence from her job, as feelings of depression and anxiety were overwhelming her. As Maggie stated,

> I am trying to bounce back, but I don't know what that looks like anymore. Susan seems to have moved on. She's back to her regular routines: work, exercise, and all that—even seeing friends. I respect her for it, but it makes it hard to connect to her.

Maggie went on to describe how she was spending her time:

> Honestly, I don't know where the days go. Suddenly, it's late afternoon and I haven't accomplished a thing. I know Susan is upset with me. Last week, she asked me to take care of some bills that needed to get paid—I still haven't done it.

Susan's frustrations with Maggie were palpable and understandable. Susan said,

> I know she's struggling, but life has to go on. I don't want to sound uncaring. I mean, I'm sorry we lost this baby too—but these things happen. I get it if Maggie needs more time off work, but she doesn't even want to hang out with friends. I'm feeling pretty alone here.

The loss and their reactions to it were creating a wedge between them.

Therapy gave Susan and Maggie a space to air all these feelings. It was important for them to be able to acknowledge each other's reactions to their loss, coming out in different patterns of grief. Maggie was demonstrating an intuitive style of grief: She felt overwhelmed by depression, retreating into herself and feeling emotionally exhausted. Susan's grief style could be seen as instrumental: She needed to connect with others, regain control by focusing on work, and avoid emotional displays. Both were grieving, but in different ways. In therapy, I explained the theory of how grief can be expressed so differently (Doka & Martin, 2011). It was also helpful to explore their reproductive story and how it went awry—especially as a same-sex couple. For Maggie, the gestational carrier, having a pregnancy loss ran counter to her sense of self as someone who was used to setting goals and achieving them. When Susan shared her experience of the loss, the dynamic between them changed. Susan began,

> You know, there's something I didn't share with you, Maggie. When we were at the hospital, the staff questioned who I was. It made me feel like I didn't belong there. Not only were we losing our baby, but at first, they weren't going to let me be with you. I was so angry; I even asked the nurse if she needed to see our wedding license.

Susan sharing this story seemed to mend the rupture that had grown between them. It was almost as if a spell had been broken. What happened over the next few weeks was a surprise to them: As Maggie started to feel better and returned to work, Susan's anxiety and sadness started to surface. As Susan observed,

> With Maggie so despondent, there was no room for my feelings. I had to counter her depression by keeping things moving. I did what I know how to do: I dove back into work—that gave me a sense of accomplishment—and got on with life. I think I bottled up my feelings to try and prop Maggie up.

Opening up and sharing their reactions to the loss, and how their feelings evolved over time, helped Maggie and Susan find the equilibrium in their relationship once again.

What this case demonstrates is the seesaw of emotions that can occur between couples—as one person starts to feel better, the other may feel worse. Person A may suggest trying again, for example, while person B wants to wait. But then when person B thinks it's a good idea to try for another pregnancy, person A may put on the brakes. This emotional seesaw happens all the time between couples, but it can also happen within an individual as well. One moment, you might want to retreat from the world; the next, you may be looking toward the future. According to Stroebe and Schut (1999), there needs to be a balance between expressing feelings about the trauma and loss that occurred and accepting the reality of how the loss has changed one's life. In other words, at the same time you may be actively grieving, you may simultaneously be attempting to rewrite your reproductive story for the future. The shifts within yourself, as well as the emotional shifts your partner may be experiencing, may seem like a lot to process. As with Maggie and Susan, patience and empathy—with yourself and with each other—can restore a sense of balance.

The previous vignettes focused on the emotional disruptions that can occur in relationships. In the next section, we'll explore sexual intimacy following a reproductive loss. Here too misunderstandings can cause flare-ups and rifts with your partner, but empathy, kindness, and caring can help bring you close together again.

INTIMACY: WHAT DOES THAT LOOK LIKE NOW?

You may be craving a warm and reassuring embrace from your partner but beyond that, the question of sexual intimacy may cause confusion and suffering. On one hand, perhaps you can't wait to have sex again—wanting to get pregnant right away to make the loss disappear. On the other hand, the idea of sex might be the furthest from your mind, with fears and worries that another loss is inevitable. What if your partner is ready and you are not? Are there differences for men and women? How do you negotiate all this?

Sex is an important element of any intimate relationship. A disruption to the sexual part of your relationship can be unsettling. One of the issues couples complain about is the loss of spontaneity when trying to conceive. Sex that is focused on conception may feel timed and mechanical and may make you wonder if you are still desired by your partner. This is true for both men and women. You may also worry that sex will be a reminder of the loss, which will trigger more grief and make you want to avoid it. You may worry that if you don't want sex, your partner will turn elsewhere. People often express concern that their partner will reject them to be with someone they can have children with, especially if they are struggling with infertility.

It may be most helpful to think of the time after pregnancy loss as an adjustment period. As we'll discuss, this is a time of healing on so many levels—from the physical to the emotional and from how you feel about yourself to the impact on your relationship, sexual and otherwise. A lot depends on the strength of your relationship before the loss and what this pregnancy meant to each of you. For some, pregnancy loss brings people closer. There may be a feeling of connectedness and tenderness with your partner as you forge ahead together after the loss. Others may struggle more, especially if the sexual aspects of their relationship feel strained. Thinking about this healing time as an adjustment period—a time to figure out the new normal and do so together—can minimize tensions.

For women and those who were assigned female at birth, this adjustment period will likely be different than for men or the nongestating partner. The most obvious difference is the physical healing of the body that must take place. From fertility treatments to the trauma of pregnancy loss, the lion's share of the burden falls on a woman's body. Women's bodies undergo massive alterations during pregnancy, which in most cases resolve after birth. Some of these alterations include hormonal changes, increased blood volume, and weight gain. A woman's anatomy changes as well, with the uterus growing and ligaments loosening to make room for a baby. These changes develop slowly throughout the pregnancy; however, with a pregnancy loss, a sudden shift occurs as a woman's body returns to her nonpregnant state. We know that women can experience postpartum mood disturbances after giving birth, but these can also occur after any pregnancy loss.

Let's consider how all this relates to sexual intimacy. The physical dimensions of pregnancy loss—the return to normal, so to speak—come with cramping and pain, blood loss, and interventions that may require surgery. Your uterus, which had been growing at a steady rate, suddenly contracts. You may produce breast milk,[2] and your breasts may become painfully engorged. You may feel

[2]Breast milk is produced as early as 16 weeks of gestation.

depressed because of not only the loss but also hormonal changes. It's not uncommon to feel sad or hopeless or to lose interest in your usual activities, including sex. Your body has been through so much, and sex may be triggering and not pleasurable—at least for now.

As with any physical trauma, your wounds need to heal. It's not as if you can see the damage as you could, say, with a broken arm. Pregnancy loss is an internal wound that takes time to heal. Many women bleed for weeks after a pregnancy loss and may not want to engage in sexual activities during that time. Historically, women have been advised to wait 3 months after an early pregnancy loss before trying to conceive. Although research has shown that trying again before 3 months does not increase the odds of another loss, some physicians still recommend this waiting period (Hurd, 2016); perhaps this has more to do with the psychological need to heal than the physical.

The question then is how do psychological factors relate to sexual intimacy for women? Erin, who had a stillborn baby at 32 weeks, described feeling depressed and overwhelmed with shame about her body. "It has been 4 months since I lost my baby," she began, "and I still look pregnant. Nothing fits. I still need to wear maternity clothes. I don't want to leave the house because of it. And I feel so unattractive. I don't want to even think about sex!" Erin is not alone. Negative body image can be a powerful determinant of anxiety and sexual dysfunction in women. In fact, many women question their femininity, wondering about their identity as a woman if they are not able to have a child.

Men may question their masculinity as well. Wayne openly described the issues he was having:

> When my wife and I were trying to conceive, we tried to maximize the right times. We even used an ovulation calculator.

> I didn't mind in the beginning. But after a few months of this, I kind of felt like a water faucet—turn it on, and then turn it off. Where was the passion in all that? After the miscarriage, when the routine started again, I began to have problems keeping an erection. I am so embarrassed to talk about this. The pressure just makes it worse.

Wayne was emotionally tired and stressed, and he had lost confidence in his body.

As discussed in this book, the impact of reproductive loss on men is often overlooked—the focus being on the woman's experience. It's important to remember that both of you are struggling in how you feel about yourself, how you feel about each other, and your sexual desires and wondering what the future will bring. In the next section, we'll discuss the importance of being able to understand what your partner is feeling after a loss, knowing that you both have your own style of coping and your own way of managing your grief. With empathy, openness, and patience, you have an opportunity to move closer in your partnership than ever before.

HOW DO WE MOVE FORWARD?

The inner workings of people when they are grieving a pregnancy loss are not simple. As discussed earlier, there is no set pattern to grief, no right way to get through it. Added to the mix is that often this is not a loss that is yours alone, but one that is shared with a significant other. Each of you will have different needs, different feelings, and different ways of handling yourself as you struggle with your new reality; your needs and feelings, as well as your partner's, will change over time. How does this affect your relationship? Is it doomed to failure, or will it grow from these experiences? What does it mean to move forward? How do you rethink your reproductive story—for yourself and with your partner?

Remember that this is an adjustment period. You are trying to figure out how to put one foot in front of the other, individually and together as a team. The loss has shattered your hopes; rebuilding new dreams out of the rubble takes time and a big dose of empathy for each other.

What exactly is empathy? *Empathy* can be described as the ability to take on another person's perspective—to see things through their eyes. There is an old saying: "You can't really understand another person until you've walked a mile in their shoes." Putting yourself in your partner's shoes can help you reflect on what they are going through, gain empathy, and adjust to your new reality. It's not easy though. What often happens in grieving a pregnancy loss is a retreat into oneself. The hurt is deeply personal. You may not be able to recognize that your partner is hurting too; in fact, you may lash out at them for not understanding you. I invite you to read on as we sample a therapy session with Clare and Travis, and witness how they were able to gain empathy and resolve differences over time.

Clare, the oldest of three, is an attorney. Travis, her husband, described her as a high achiever and admired her ability to act in the defense of her clients. Travis, warm and sensitive, is a children's book author and illustrator. He was excited about finally starting their own family. "What a thrill it will be to read to our kids! It's something I've always dreamed about," he said. Unfortunately, this snippet of his reproductive story was cut short. I began seeing them in therapy several months after Clare and Travis made the heartbreaking decision to terminate their pregnancy because of a condition known as Edwards syndrome or trisomy 18. This condition occurs when the developing fetus has three copies of chromosome 18 instead of the normal two. The couple had been advised that the odds of a full-term pregnancy were slim; if their baby did survive birth, she would have multiple health problems and probably live for only a week or so. The decision seemed logical but was fraught with guilt, especially for Clare. Her religious background, which had not played a huge role in her adult life, suddenly was more prevalent. It made her doubt herself and question the body of scientific knowledge she was presented with. "It's her body and ultimately her decision," Travis said. "I didn't want to tell Clare what to do, but there was really only one logical path forward."

After the termination, Clare continued to express doubts that they did the right thing. "What if the doctors were wrong?" she tearfully cried. She was wracked with worries about what other people would think of them, concerned that she would be accused of having had an abortion. She told people that she had a miscarriage, so as not to be judged, and she begged Travis to do the same. Having to lie about their experience went against Travis's moral code. "I'm going along with this for Clare, but I don't agree with her, and I'm actually pretty upset by keeping it a secret." Calling their loss a miscarriage added to his pain. He felt stifled as he was unable to talk with others about the reality of their trauma.

When Clare and Travis began couple's therapy, things were not going well. Clare was not her usual outgoing self. She had withdrawn from most of the activities she had enjoyed in the past, especially those that involved seeing other people. Travis was frustrated and not sure what to do. He was concerned that this was the way life was going to be from now on, asking, "Is she ever going to get beyond this?" A deep chasm was forming between them with no bridge to connect them. While the rift was rooted in their reproductive loss, it had been playing out in daily life ever since. To bridge this gap, it was important for them to understand how deeply their loss shook and challenged their basic core beliefs, recognize each other's divergent grief styles, and agree to try to build a new pathway forward.

It was clear that Clare and Travis's pregnancy demise veered far from the expectations they had. They were in accord on this point, but how they were each managing their grief was diverging. I asked if they had done anything to memorialize their loss. Travis talked about some drawings he was working on: "I've been thinking about trying to incorporate all this into a new book. Maybe something that could help other parents talk to kids about loss."

"What?" Clare asked with surprise. "Why haven't you told me about this?"

"Honestly," Travis began, "I was a little worried about how you would respond. Like you'd think I was going public, and that would make you upset."

Clare was silent for a moment and then replied, "What's making me upset is that you've been keeping a secret from me. I thought we were trying to communicate more, not hide things from each other."

Here, again, you likely recognize the pattern of POSR, in which one partner (Travis, in this case) held back their feelings for fear of upsetting the other partner (Clare). Travis's effort to protect Clare by not telling her about writing about their loss, however, made Clare more unsettled with the growing gap between them. When we talked about POSR as a common reaction between couples, Travis agreed that it wasn't the best idea to keep his drawings and ideas from Clare. "Honestly, though," he countered, "you've been so withdrawn that I don't know how to approach you. When I've tried to bring things up—I'm even afraid to bring this up here—you've made it clear that it's off limits." Clare was silent, but her eyes began to well. It was clear that each partner was dealing with their grief in their own way. At this point, they did not feel connected; rather, they were struggling alone. I intervened:

> What if you were to let each other know you wanted, or needed, to talk about something? Kind of prepared each other, maybe asking, "Is this a good time to talk?" If it is, well then you can have a discussion. If not, maybe you could set up another time?

"Well, there is something I want to bring up," Travis began, "and I wonder if this would be a good time to bring it up." He turned to Clare and asked, "Would this be a good time to talk about your cousin's wedding?" He turned to me and said, "We had an argument about this yesterday." By asking Clare about this topic, he was making sure she would be willing to engage in it. It wasn't approached with anger or resentment, giving Clare some control over accepting or rejecting this conversation. Clare filled in details:

> My cousin, Rita, is getting married and if we're going, we need to buy plane tickets and make hotel reservations. Travis is upset because we haven't made our travel plans yet. I just don't know if I want to go.

"This is so not like her," Travis said, shaking his head and turning to me. "Rita is her favorite cousin; the whole family will be there. In the past, Clare would have made these arrangements as soon as Rita told us the news. And it's now just weeks away."

"But you don't understand, Travis," Clare said. "I was supposed to be in the wedding party. I even had a maternity dress made. What am I supposed to wear now? I can't stand up in front of all those people—I just can't."

At first, Travis was dismissive. He thought, how important could a dress be? Why couldn't Clare wear something else? As we talked more, however, he began to understand that the dress was emblematic of the loss and of the deep shame and guilt she felt. She worried that people would talk about them, wonder what really happened, and then pity them. This was all too much for her to bear. Instead of talking to Travis about her concerns because she didn't think he would understand, Clare withdrew more. Her withdrawal caused Travis to become more irritated, making her withdraw even more. This cycle, which can happen frequently between a couple, was deepening the divide between them.

Pointing out this pattern was essential. Understanding the downward spiral this cycle was creating—and its interference with their ability to move forward—was a step toward bridging the gap. "I'm wondering," I began, "if there is a way to manage your attendance at Rita's wedding. Aside from not going at all, can you think of how you might handle it together?"

"I think if I were in Clare's shoes—or in this case, her dress," Travis joked, "I'm wondering if Clare could get out of being in the wedding party altogether? I mean, is that the only way you can show your love for Rita?" he asked. "That way, you're not on display, you can wear what you want, and you can just interact with the family as you feel like. What do you think about that, hon?"

"I had actually thought about this, but I was afraid Rita would take it the wrong way," Clare said. I noted that her pattern of withdrawing from emotional confrontation was repeating itself with Rita as well.

"What if we wrote her a note together?" asked Travis, offering a solution. He continued:

> I could even do a special drawing for it—and explain that we are struggling. Please note, I am emphasizing *we* here. We can let her know how happy we are to be coming, but that it would better for *us* not to be in the wedding party. Given who Rita is, I don't think she would be upset. She'd totally understand that we may need to take breaks from the celebration.

Before we ended the session for that day, I wanted to underscore Clare and Travis's ability to work together and how they found empathy for each other. They were not each other's enemy. In fact, if they found themselves angry or retreating from each other, could they reflect on the underlying issue that was upsetting them? Could they let each other know they needed to talk? Finding empathy was not just about this upcoming wedding but was paramount to all aspects of their communication. It would allow them to move forward together whenever conflicts or major decisions arose. Exercise 5.1 further describes the importance of empathy and tenderness in relationships.

As we'll address in Chapter 7, one of the most difficult issues facing couples is often the decision to try again—opening old wounds and fears. Having a solid foundation in your relationship, one where you can allow for differences in grief by walking in your partner's shoes, will help you traverse the bumpy road ahead.

EXERCISE 5.1. Developing Empathy and Tenderness

As you have been reading through the examples of couples who are grieving and trying to reckon with their pregnancy loss, no doubt you have been thinking about your own relationship. Take a moment and ask yourself the following questions:

- What are some things that make you concerned about your partner? How worried are you about their commitment to you and the relationship?
- Are there things you would like to talk to your partner about but that you are holding back on?
- Are you worried your partner does not understand how you are feeling?
- What are you afraid of? Are you concerned that your partner is judging you? Are you worried what other people might be thinking—that somehow you are at fault?

EXERCISE 5.1. Developing Empathy and Tenderness (*Continued*)

- Can you list five things you need from your partner right now? Can you let them know some of the things you need?
- What do you think your partner needs from you? Can you let them know that you are willing to listen?

Oftentimes, reflecting on your own needs—and then giving that exact thing to your partner—can break down the barriers that are separating you.

Let's go back to the image of a boxing ring. You and your partner are sitting in your opposing corners. The referee asks you to come out and shake hands before the fight. What if you took off the boxing gloves and gave each other a hug instead? Often, what people need most during and after a reproductive loss is tenderness.

It would be wonderful if both of you could approach each other with kindness and affection at the same time. If this doesn't happen—and you find yourself resentfully waiting for your partner to know what you need—perhaps you can initiate it. It's likely your partner is craving the same thing from you. It is impossible to read someone else's mind but if you reflect on your own feelings, then it's a safe bet that your partner is grieving as well.

Sometimes squeezing your partner's hand is all that is needed to nonverbally connect. The words—the discussion of feelings and what lies ahead—can follow. You can model what you need in your grief by taking these small actions. The more you are able to give your partner what you also need, the more you will be able to receive it as well. It is worth trying this out; hopefully it will help construct a new foundation of intimacy for both of you to move forward.

SUMMARY

Grief following a pregnancy loss is incredibly difficult. Your whole world has been upended, and you are trying your best to cope with overwhelming pain and loss. To complicate matters, your partner is also grieving. Although it is the same loss, the effects on each of you, how you grieve, and how you manage your feelings may look nothing alike. Because the outward expressions of grief can be so vastly different, misunderstandings between partners often occur.

Reading this chapter hopefully shed light on the many ways people express grief. As stated earlier, there is no one right way to get through the pain of a pregnancy loss. Increasing self-knowledge of your own expression of grief and how it may differ from your partner's will help decrease any confusion or misinterpretations that may arise. Learning to approach your partner with kindness and love—especially at times of great distress—can help fill the gaping hole that your loss has caused.

In Chapter 1, I discussed the ripple effect that reproductive losses can have, starting with the impact on you and your self-esteem, moving outward to the ways in which the loss affects the many different relationships in your life (see Figure 1.1). In this chapter, the focus was on your most intimate relationship—that of you and your partner—who have shared this loss and are trying to manage your grief both individually and together. In Chapter 6, we will move into how to manage other relationships—with family, friends, work colleagues, and the child-centric world we live in. Chapter 6 also highlights the emotional land mines that you may want to, and need to, avoid. It discusses coping with the holidays, handling events such as baby showers, and anticipating what it might be like when you return to work. Throughout, the chapter offers practical advice on how to cope as you navigate life following your loss.

CHAPTER 6

I FEEL INVISIBLE: COPING IN A CHILD-CENTRIC WORLD

It's inevitable: You run into someone you haven't seen in a while, and they look down and see you're not pregnant. You attend a family gathering, and you feel people tiptoeing around you. You go shopping at the grocery store or to the mall, and it seems that everyone else is pregnant! You watch a movie and sure enough, a character is dealing with infertility. Someone you have just met asks, "Do you have any kids?" You go back to work after a leave of absence; most people know what you've been through, but there always seems to be that one person who cheerfully asks, "How's the baby?" These kinds of situations arise time and again.

When you are experiencing a pregnancy loss, you may feel invisible and out of place in a world that is so focused on family and children. The emotional land mines you have to navigate are all around; sometimes you can predict them, but often they take you by surprise. You may think a particular situation is safe, but then a comment is made or an invitation to a baby shower arrives in your inbox and you are plunged into despair. Because of all this, it would be understandable if you wanted to isolate more; but at the same time, this is when you most need support and connection. While there really is no way to avoid the challenges inherent in a society that focuses on family, the question is how do you handle them? This chapter offers practical advice and strategies for how to cope with the world.

Here is a note of caution: Having ways of effectively traversing uncomfortable situations does not eliminate the pain you may experience. You will still feel it, and your grief will not disappear. The suggestions offered here are simply helpful tips to ease you through these instances. However, don't be surprised if your sadness or anger reemerges.

Although advice is offered in this chapter, there are many ways to cope and manage these stressful circumstances. Figuring out what works best for you is key. Exercise 6.1 describes how to create an emotional toolbox to help you manage these situations. In the following sections, we'll focus on a variety of common stressful situations and discuss ways to navigate them.

EXERCISE 6.1. Creating a Toolbox

Having an emotional toolbox at hand, in which you create a collection of things to say or develop escape routes from difficult situations, can make difficult social situations easier to manage. Having something planned can be like prepping for a major presentation: It helps you to not be caught off guard. You might think about it like preparing to act in a play. You rehearse your lines repeatedly so they come to you naturally when you are on stage. As you read through the different vignettes presented in this chapter, it might be helpful to keep a list of the things you might say or do. These will become the tools you can reach for. One woman described feeling comforted by having "imaginary pieces of paper in my pocket, each with a different message on them, that I can pull out whenever I need one."

COPING WITH HOLIDAYS

From Halloween through the New Year, we are inundated with events that are child focused. This is all well and good, except when you are grieving a reproductive loss. Whatever your perspective on these holidays, it has probably changed—at least for now. As you read through this section, take note of tools you might add to your emotional toolbox. Although we focus on holiday gatherings here, you can easily substitute any occasion (weddings, birthday parties, dinner parties, etc.) that brings people together to socialize and celebrate.

Jasmine: Holiday Traditions

Thanksgiving had always been Jasmine's favorite holiday. Although her siblings and their partners were spread out across the country, they all came together for Thanksgiving. It was the one holiday that her family had hosted for years, expanding it to include extended family and friends, with anywhere from 30 to 40 people in attendance. They would clear the living room of furniture and set up tables and chairs to create one gigantic dining table to accommodate everyone. Jasmine's job, aside from helping in the kitchen, was to set the table and create the seating arrangement, trying to strategically place people for lively conversation. Food was obviously the highlight of the day, but the family's other tradition was to go around the table and have each guest say what they were thankful for that year. Some speeches were funny, and others were heartfelt and personal. Jasmine always looked forward to this part of the dinner for the chance to hear other's reflections—their stories—on the passing year and on the future.

After much contemplation, Jasmine decided to have a baby on her own. At 36 years old, she was concerned about waiting much longer; without letting her family know, she used a sperm donor to become pregnant. She had been hoping to share the news of her pregnancy as people gave their thanks around the table. She would have been just past her first trimester, the perfect time to announce it to the crowd. Unfortunately, she had a blighted ovum, also known as an *anembryonic pregnancy*, which occurs when the gestational sac and placenta grow but the embryo doesn't develop in the sac. About a month ago, Jasmine's pregnancy ended in a miscarriage. While she was once thrilled to tell everyone her news, now the idea of standing up at the table and proclaiming what she was thankful for filled her with dread. What was she supposed to say? How was she going to handle this? Jasmine's first thought was to not go, but it would be strange if she wasn't present. Could she say she wasn't feeling well and vanish into a bedroom? That would probably create more questions and draw more attention to her than she wanted. And how do you not feel well at dinner but return wanting to try all the desserts? The truth was, she just wasn't up for celebrating at all.

Let's look at some of Jasmine's options and consider what you might do in a similar situation. There is always the possibility of not attending at all, as Jasmine considered initially. This is true for any celebratory gathering that brings together a group of people—be it a wedding, bridal shower, birthday party, or any other event, large or small. Depending on the situation, it really is okay to make up an excuse and not go. For example, let's say that a friend has invited you to their bridal shower. If this is a very close friendship, you might let your friend know the truth—that for now you are not feeling sociable. You might even suggest that the two of you get together privately instead. This approach lets your friend know that you would still like to spend time together but not in a group for the time being.

If you don't feel comfortable telling the host what you are going through, how else could you handle it? If you feel like it is important to make an appearance, one option is to arrive late and leave early if feasible. If you are going to an event with your partner, you both can make a pact to stick together and support each other. If one of you is having a difficult time socializing, perhaps the other can step in. Likewise, talking with your partner beforehand and establishing a signal to alert each other that it's time to leave can help. What if one of you is having a great time and the other isn't? Is the possible friction between you worth staying at a party longer? Agreeing ahead of time about your strategy to leave, even if one of you would rather stay, emphasizes that you are in this together—this is such an important message when you are dealing with a reproductive loss.

Another helpful strategy is to excuse yourself from a conversation that feels overwhelming. The call of nature, so to speak, has saved many people from awkward, uncomfortable conversations. For example, if your Great Aunt Mildred corners you and asks when you are going to have kids, you can politely say, "Oh, would you excuse me? I was just heading to the restroom." In fact, going to the restroom and locking the door—whether your bladder is calling or not—is a way to take a moment for yourself. You can take a deep breath, center yourself, and even cry before you return to fend off Great Aunt Mildred. One woman, when confronted by her nosy relative, said, "Are you trying to find out about my sex life?" That ended the conversation quickly! Talking with your host beforehand if possible, having a signal with your partner, and strategically going to the restroom are all strategies to include in your emotional toolbox.

Let's get back to the specifics of Jasmine's situation. How was she going to handle all the people at Thanksgiving, and what was she going to say when it was her turn to stand up and give thanks? Backing out was not an option, nor was it possible to arrive late; she was staying with her parents, and her help with all the preparations was expected. After the meal, it might be possible for Jasmine to disappear for a bit, which did bring her some relief; that small modicum of control was helpful. As for her message of thanks, she decided to keep it very generic and simple and said, "I'm so thankful for being able to spend another Thanksgiving with you all."

One thing that made Jasmine's situation so difficult was that she was one of the hosts of the Thanksgiving celebration. Here is a word of advice: Even if you have always hosted a particular event, you might consider letting someone else step up and do it this time. When you are the host, there is no way you can escape. You can't show up late or leave early. While the preparations may feel like a good distraction, the reality is that it may prove to be too much. If it is possible to change the venue to someone else's home or hold the festivities in a restaurant this year, you can still participate but take some of the pressure off.

ANSWERING THE QUESTION "DO YOU HAVE KIDS?"

During conversations at social gatherings, people often talk about their children. Whether people talk about their children with pride or frustration or just say that they need to head out to relieve the babysitter, they are a common topic that you need to be prepared for. Invariably, the question will turn to you: "Do you have kids?" You might even be asked not if you have kids but rather how many, with the assumption being that of course you have children and more than one.

I remember an incident that occurred at a party I was attending. A gentleman whom I had never met before asked if I had kids. When I told him, yes, I had a son, he loudly proclaimed, "Just one? You people think having an only child is a good thing! Where I come from, we always have big families!" He knew nothing about me and had no idea of my history of loss, nor was I at all interested in sharing it with him. I smiled, backed away, and left as soon as I could. I am sharing this with you because these kinds of interactions can happen unexpectedly and take you by surprise. Having your toolbox at the ready can really be of help.

How could I have handled that situation differently? I could have told the man the truth. "Yes, I have an only child, but having just one child wasn't by choice." But I was so taken aback and, as I said, I did not want to engage with him. I have known other people who have said, "No, I don't have any *living* children," when asked if they had children and then went on to inform the person of their circumstances. It really depends on the situation and if you feel safe talking with the person about your loss. I know of one woman who bluntly said, "Yes, but my baby died," and left the other person squirming uncomfortably. It did end the conversation.

What are some other ways to deal with the question of whether you have kids? You can say, "No, I don't have children" or "Not yet," and leave it at that. If the conversation becomes more probing, you can always rely on the restroom trick and excuse yourself. If you decide not to talk about your loss, it is helpful to have two simultaneous conversations: one outward, and the other in your head. The outward conversation, which denies having children or only counts those who are living, differs from the inward dialogue, which takes that moment to remember your story and the attachment and connection with your baby. There are times after a loss, even years later, when people will outwardly reply with the number of children who are living while they inwardly remember the real count.

HANDLING DINNER PARTIES

Sometimes larger gatherings of people are easier to navigate than smaller, more intimate ones. It's easier to get lost in the crowd at a bigger event and easier to move from one conversation to another. Dinner parties can prove to be more anxiety provoking; you may feel more put on the spot to engage, and there may be fewer avenues of escape.

Lydia: Self-Talk

Lydia, a 32-year-old graphic designer, was invited to a girl's night out with six other women, and she decided to go. She thought it would be good for her; her husband encouraged her to get out of the house and get out of the rut she had been in since her ectopic pregnancy. The other women didn't know about Lydia's loss, and she was hopeful that the conversation wouldn't focus on babies.

The women were seated at a long table at a restaurant. Lydia squeezed into a spot in the middle with her back against a wall. As the waiter took their drink orders, one woman smiled slyly and remarked that she wasn't drinking. It took but a second for everyone else to remark and squeal with delight—everyone, that is, except Lydia. "My heart sank as I realized where the evening was headed. I also realized that all the other women had kids, except for me and another woman sitting across from me. Was she feeling the same way I was?" Lydia wondered. "At least she wasn't trapped between two other women and a wall!" she said angrily. "Let's just say it was not a great night."

Lydia's foray into a social situation did not go well. She tried to engage with the other child-free woman at the table and tried unsuccessfully to change the subject, but the conversation was dominated by the pregnant woman's due date, the baby's gender, how the woman was feeling, and all her preparations for her first baby. One tool that Lydia stored in her portable emotional toolbox was *self-talk*. In essence, self-talk is an inner dialogue you have with yourself that can boost your self-esteem. Self-talk is a way to stop your inner critic—that negative voice in your head that can take over. Here is how to use self-talk:

1. Remind yourself that your reaction of anxiety, despair, sadness, or hostility is perfectly logical given the circumstances. In this case, Lydia's feelings of being trapped were totally understandable. She could have gone down the path of thinking of herself as an utter failure, but she was able to short-circuit those thoughts.

2. Self-talk can remind you of all the positive aspects of yourself. At the dinner, Lydia was able to call to mind her solid relationship with her husband and the current project she was excited to be working on, and she counted the many other things she had going for herself. Talking to herself about her strengths and accomplishments reminded Lydia that wanting a family was only one piece of her life.
3. Keep things in perspective. Lydia's self-talk included remembering that this gathering was not infinite and would end soon. The dinner would be over in an hour or so. She told herself that getting through this—and practicing strategies that emphasized the positive rather than what was missing—would make the next event easier.

MANAGING BABY SHOWERS

Does it seem as if everyone around you is pregnant or has just had a baby? When you are of reproductive age, you likely have friends and family—brothers, sisters, cousins—who are in the same cohort. It's to be expected that your peers will all be thinking of starting a family right around the same time that you are. In Chapter 3, we talked about assumptions we have about pregnancy; the assumption of being on the same pregnancy timeline as everyone else is natural.

What goes hand in hand with having a baby? Baby showers. You may find yourself inundated with invitations to celebrate the upcoming birth of someone else's baby. Their good fortune may be incredibly painful for you. It's not that you don't want them to have this moment of joy; it's just that you may not want to join in the festivities. That is perfectly understandable. Watching prospective parents open cute baby gifts could be agonizing. In fact, based on your experience of pregnancy loss, you may be very superstitious about any celebration before the birth of a child. You may be thinking, "What if something goes wrong?"

How do you deal with the pressure to attend? We previously discussed strategies to manage holidays and other social gatherings, but baby showers may be too stressful. Please hear this: It's okay not to go! You are not a bad friend if you don't show up. How you manage the situation depends on your relationship with the parents-to-be. One strategy is to talk with them openly and honestly: Let them know why you can't make an appearance, and perhaps find a time to meet and celebrate privately. Another option is to say that you had a previous engagement; this little white lie can be forgiven based on your current psychological and emotional state. You can send a gift or order something through a registry if available, expressing your support and congratulations. Sometimes even going to a website to order a gift can be too painful; gift cards work just as well, and they allow you to avoid all of the baby paraphernalia.

THINKING ABOUT MOTHER'S DAY AND FATHER'S DAY

Of all the holidays throughout the year, Mother's Day and Father's Day, which celebrate and honor parenthood, can be the hardest of them all. These special days are reminders that the children who should be with you—running around, playing with toys, snuggling with books—are absent. These holidays also hit hard at your sense of identity: Are you a parent or not? As discussed throughout this volume, you are a parent psychologically even if you don't have the children to show for it. It is so important for you to acknowledge that you were the best parent you could be given the circumstance. Your love is evident, measured by the grief you have experienced.

The question remains: How do you handle Mother's Day and Father's Day? Maybe you and your partner decide to turn off your electronic devices for the day, get out into nature, and go off the grid.

Maybe you decide to spend time together with other people who don't have children. If you usually celebrate with your own parents, the choice is yours as to whether you want to do so. You can always explain to them that you are just not up for it this time. Whatever you choose to do, treat yourself and your partner with kindness and care. Recognize that you are both hurting. You need to give each other as much support as you can.

NAVIGATING HURTFUL WORDS OR AVOIDANCE

It is inevitable that someone will offer advice or what they think are words of comfort. Some remarks, such as "Don't worry, you can have another" or "It was for the best," speak to the awkwardness that other people feel around pregnancy losses. You may very well be able to conceive again and have a child, but there are no guarantees of that happening. Also, you cannot simply replace one child with another. It is not another child that you want; it is the child you are grieving. Likewise, any pregnancy loss is not for the best; rather, it's just the opposite. We understand the meaning of these remarks, which are not meant to be mean-spirited, but they are clumsy attempts to console. What is said from a place of well-meaning can be received as grossly insensitive and hurtful. It can also feel tactless and unkind if someone avoids talking about your loss. What they may perceive as being helpful ("Let's just move on and pretend this didn't happen") can feel just as painful. Next, we will look at some cases where helpful words (or silence) felt like a knife stab, and we will discuss how people handled the situation.

Lauren: Ruptures in Relationships

Lauren, 38, and her husband, Paul, 42, had been struggling to conceive for several years. With the advice of their reproductive specialist, they decided to pursue family building using an egg donor. Making this shift in their reproductive story was not easy. They were grieving the loss of using Lauren's eggs; at the same time, they were excited about the possibility of becoming parents, knowing their chances would be much greater using the eggs of a younger donor. To give you an idea, the odds of getting pregnant for a healthy 30-year-old are 20% each month of trying; by age 40, they are less than 5% each cycle (American Society for Reproductive Medicine, 2012). Once Lauren and Paul decided to use an egg donor, they were faced with the daunting task of choosing one. Paul wanted to find someone who resembled Lauren, thinking that would limit people's questions. Although Lauren agreed, most important to her were the donor's health, education, and interests. The more Lauren and Paul accepted this path forward, the more they agreed that using a donor was not something they should feel ashamed of nor did they want to keep it a secret. They were proud of their decision, and they told family and friends that they would be part of a new generation of parents.

The search went on until Lauren and Paul finally found a young woman who seemed like a good match. They were excited to move forward with in vitro fertilization (IVF) using the egg donor. Paul's sperm was combined with the donor's eggs in the lab; they were delighted to have five embryos from the procedure. The next step was to transfer the embryos (one at a time) into Lauren's uterus. Their hopes dimmed, however, after two transfers were not successful. Although they still had three more possible transfers, their hopes faltered. As Lauren and Paul told the people close to them about the failed cycles, the interactions were, for the most part, caring and supportive. Some people's reactions were, as Lauren put it, "mind-boggling," leaving Lauren and Paul to wonder if they could continue a relationship with them. Lauren noted one close friend, Kim, who essentially disappeared on her:

> When I told Kim about our losses, she said she was sorry and then told me about some upcoming travel she had planned. We agreed to see each other when she returned. But then, nothing. Radio silence. I've reached out a few times and never got a call or text back. I'm not sure how to handle this.

Because Kim wasn't responding to her calls or texts, Lauren chose to send her a handwritten letter—a rarity in communication these days and sure to get her attention. A letter would allow Kim time to think about a response and not be put on the spot. Lauren wrote about her feelings, and she acknowledged how difficult it can be to understand that a failed IVF cycle was a pregnancy loss. Lauren attempted to educate Kim and let her know how hurt she was by Kim ghosting her. Lauren also asked Kim if something else was going on in Kim's life that was troubling her. Even though part of Lauren was angry with Kim, she turned it around and tried to see it from Kim's perspective.

Lauren was also struggling with Paul's sister, Bonnie. We should note that Bonnie had two biological children and had no problems with either of her pregnancies. Bonnie had been supportive of Lauren and Paul throughout their journey, which made Bonnie's comment even more disconcerting. Lauren cried as she shared the following:

> I know my mouth was hanging open when Bonnie said, "At least it wasn't yours." I had to ask her to repeat herself because I was so dumbfounded. Bonnie said, "Well, it was somebody else's egg." As if that made a difference! So, here is another relationship that I don't know how to handle. I don't want this to cause a rift in the family, but right now I need some space from her.

In any of these difficult situations, it is important to know that you don't have to do it alone. Consider this—reaching out to someone you can rely on and talk things through with—another tool in that growing emotional toolbox. Often, this person will be your partner, but it could also be a close friend, a family member, or your therapist. Lauren initially didn't want to burden Paul or cause him to think negatively about his sister. The more Lauren thought about it, though, the more she knew she needed his support. Paul too was aghast when he heard what his sister had said. Together they reached out to Bonnie to share their feelings.

Sadly, there are times when relationships cannot be repaired. It is true that life crises can bring out the very best—and the very worst—in people. We can be taken by surprise and deeply disappointed when the people we thought we could count on are just not available. This is another layer of loss that reproductive traumas can unveil. Yet we can be just as surprised to find others in our midst who unexpectedly rise to the occasion. They seem to know what to do, and they know exactly what we need. A stronger bond may develop than before, and for that we can be thankful.

TALKING WITH CHILDREN

Grappling with the death of a baby is hard enough as an adult, but think about what it must be like to understand it through the eyes of a child. If you already have a child or children, they are experiencing the death of their sibling. Their understanding of pregnancy loss will differ, depending on the their age. Likewise, how you talk to them about it needs to be age appropriate. Regardless of where they are developmentally, children will have many questions and concerns. Parents need to be prepared to talk repeatedly about the loss with their grieving child, even as they themselves are grieving. Questions may arise unexpectedly and can trigger your own thoughts and feelings as you struggle to guide and reassure your child or children.

Mollie and Ben: Comforting a Sibling

Here is a case example of how Mollie and Ben discussed their loss with their 3-year-old son, Eli. Mollie was pregnant with her second child, a girl; Eli was so excited about having a baby sister to play with. Mollie encouraged Eli to draw pictures for his sister's arrival, and they hung them up as they prepared the nursery. At 37 weeks of pregnancy, Mollie stopped feeling fetal movement. She had been monitoring kick counts and when they subsided, she knew something was not right. A visit to the hospital labor and delivery department confirmed the worst: Their daughter, Carolyn, had died.

In their grief, Mollie and Ben were also concerned about Eli. They struggled with knowing what to say and how to talk with Eli about Carolyn's death. Did he understand what had happened? In simple terms, they told him that Carolyn's body just stopped working and that it wasn't anybody's fault; this was important for Eli to hear, because it is common for young children to think they did something wrong. For example, if at any point Eli had thought about not wanting a sister (e.g., maybe wishing for a brother instead), he may have believed he caused her death. Mollie and Ben talked about how bad things sometimes happen. They tried their best to reassure Eli that he was safe and that they were still a family that loved and cared for each other.

Carolyn's funeral was held a week later. Family and friends were there to offer support and love. As one might expect, Eli received a great deal of attention, although he wasn't sure what it all meant. He understood that Carolyn was going to be in a place called a cemetery and, in his 3-year-old concept of the world, hoped she would be able to come home soon. He also knew how sad his mom and dad were and wanted somehow to make it better for them.

At the funeral, Ben was holding Eli and heard a female friend of the family say, "You need to be happy that you have Eli." What did that mean? Eli could tell Ben was angry as he felt his dad's grip on him grow stronger; Eli also felt sad and confused as he watched his mother's eyes fill with tears. His parents quickly turned and walked away. Later, when they were back at home, Eli asked, "What did that lady mean?" Were they not happy to have Eli? Did he do something wrong? Their first response was to make sure Eli knew that the woman was not being mean. "Sometimes grown-ups say things they think are going to make you feel better, but they say it in a way that makes you feel worse," Mollie began. "She was trying to take some of our sadness away by telling us how wonderful you are," Ben continued. Mollie added, "I'm so glad we're talking about this, Eli. I bet this is all very hard to understand. Sometimes it's hard for me and dad to understand too, but you can always ask us questions."

"You know," Ben said, "you can still draw pictures for Carolyn. We can make a special book of them so you can remember her. You can let her know about all your adventures." Here, Ben was instinctively promoting the idea of continuing bonds—that Carolyn would always be in their hearts. Ben added, "Just know that we love you to the moon and back!" Eli giggled, as this was one of his favorite things to say. "Yeah, to the moon and back!" he repeated, and ran off to play.

REFLECTING ON ANNIVERSARY DATES

Your calendar once may have held reminders of family birthdays and anniversaries but is now filled with other significant dates. Now your calendar tracks what should have been your due date, along with the date of your loss or the death of your baby. These anniversary dates are not celebratory but are times of reflection and remembrance. They are now forever etched into your year. Sadly, these dates may add to feeling invisible and alone; it often happens that other people don't remember these days as significant, and that can hurt. As you read on, you will see some ways people have handled these painful times. But just as there is no one right way to grieve, ongoing remembrances are unique to each person.

Jordan: Taking Time to Remember

"It happens without fail," Jordan said. "I think it might be the change in the light at this time of year. I may not even be aware of the calendar, but at the beginning of March, I get a pang of sadness." It had been 5 years since Jordan's son, Aaron, was born still. She has since given birth to her daughter, Cassie, now 3. Jordan explained how she remembers the anniversary:

> The first year after Aaron's birth and death, I remember thinking I could just throw myself into work. But that whole week before the anniversary date, I was a mess. Now I make sure to take the day off from work. It's my day to do whatever I need to do, my day to honor Aaron. Having Cassie is a wonderful reminder not to take things for granted. It has definitely gotten easier with time.

It is not uncommon to think you can power through these hot-button dates, but more often they are charged with emotion. We frequently look back to the previous year and reexamine the trauma. With each passing year, you may again look at the prior year; the memories of how you honored your baby each year build as your reproductive story morphs over time. For Jordan, creating a time and space to remember Aaron, while celebrating Cassie, has developed into a yearly ritual.

Janelle: Dealing With Self-Imposed Expectations

Janelle shared the following in regard to her miscarriage:

> My miscarriage was 6 months ago. I was really hoping to be pregnant before my due date—or what should have been my due date. It's coming up now, and I feel like I've got a double whammy of loss to deal with.

Janelle was struggling with her sense of self. The miscarriage made her feel damaged, as if she wasn't fully a woman. For Janelle, getting pregnant again before her due date would symbolize that she was whole again. The pressure she felt to prove her worth as a woman was accentuating her stress. Eliminating the self-imposed deadline of getting pregnant by her due date was essential to decreasing her anxiety. As Janelle worked through the double whammy (as she described it), it was important for her to remind herself repeatedly that there was more to her than being pregnant and becoming a mom. As she stated, "It's hard to honor the things about myself that are good—my relationships, my career, the things I enjoy—because there's a huge hole where a baby should be. I'm trying as best as I can."

Sharon and Mark: Reminding Others of What You Need

Sharon and Mark now have a 3-year-old daughter, but their path to parenthood was not easy. "You would never know to look at her," Mark said of Sharon. "She swims 5 days a week and is totally fit!" Sharon, athletic and slender with long curly black hair, got tears in her eyes and said sarcastically, "Yeah, totally fit until my blood pressure shot up to ridiculously high numbers." Mark grabbed her hand and continued, "We did everything we could, but we had to terminate that pregnancy. We couldn't take a risk with Sharon's health.

Terminating that pregnancy was the only route forward. And afterward, her blood pressure went back to normal!"

Sharon and Mark's loss had brought up so many unknowns. What was the risk should Sharon get pregnant again? Should they pursue a different route to become parents? And if so, what would be the best path forward: surrogacy or adoption? They decided to pursue surrogacy because they would be able to use Sharon's eggs to create embryos. Their daughter's birth was celebrated by both sets of grandparents with utter joy; all doted on her and showered her with attention. While it was wonderful for all that Sharon and Mark were now parents, acknowledgment of their first pregnancy loss was still important. Sharon and Mark felt it was such an important event in their lives that they did not want it to be forgotten, especially by their own parents.

Mark's parents seemed not to remember or acknowledge their pregnancy loss. It was as if it had never happened. Why bring up something painful, they thought, when there was so much joy around having their granddaughter? This was in contrast with Sharon's parents, who sent a card and called each year on the date of their termination. While it is true that many people forget the date, they do not necessarily forget the event.

Not acknowledging the loss, however, hurt Sharon and Mark's feelings. If you find yourself in a similar situation, you can always just ask. It may be that grandparents, who are grieving as well, are concerned about bringing it up—not wanting to hurt you, their own child. This was, in fact, the case for Mark's parents. They were trying to be protective in not bringing up sad memories, so they chose to ignore the anniversary date. Remember the phenomenon of partner-oriented self-regulation (POSR)? POSR is where one person in the relationship suppresses their own feelings to protect the other person (Stroebe et al., 2013). In this case, we can see POSR happening between parents and grandparents: Mark's parents were trying to protect Sharon and Mark from negative feelings by not acknowledging the date of their pregnancy demise, but this was causing Sharon and Mark pain and discomfort. Talking about these dynamics, when possible, can help clear up misunderstandings. As simple as it sounds, talking about things is another tool in the emotional toolbox. In this case, by letting Mark's parents know that a simple recognition was all Sharon and Mark needed, the connection in the family was restored.

RETURNING TO WORK

After a loss, returning to work can feel like one of the most daunting transitions. Numerous factors influence decisions about returning to work. Here are some examples:

- What type of loss have you experienced?
- Does your place of employment have bereavement leave? If so, does that include reproductive losses?
- Do you work from home, or do you need to be present at the workplace?
- What are the physical demands of your work? Are you on your feet all day, or do you sit at a desk?
- Do you enjoy your work?
- Do you have to return to work (e.g., perhaps for financial reasons) before you want to?
- Do coworkers know of your pregnancy?
- How do you manage conversations about your pregnancy and loss with others?

As we delve into these questions, one challenge we will note is the sense of returning to normal that work implies. Regardless of the loss you have experienced, going back to work represents moving on with life. For some, diving into work is a good distraction. It can be a reminder of all your strengths and the multiple dimensions of your life. Others may just not feel ready, especially if they are having difficulty maintaining focus and concentration. Obviously, you have been changed by your pregnancy loss; your reproductive story has moved in a direction that you didn't anticipate. You are recuperating physically and psychologically, which is perhaps the most difficult task of all. Think about it: What was your last day of work like before your loss? You knew you were pregnant, with new beginnings and possibilities opening for you—regardless of whether others knew. Now the picture looks very different. Your grief has taken over, and you have been changed forever.

The type of loss you have had will likely dictate the amount of time off you need. If you've had a miscarriage, you may be physically ready to return to work after just a few days. You may need a longer leave of absence after an ectopic pregnancy or stillbirth. The Family and Medical Leave Act (FMLA) states that employees may take leave to recover from a pregnancy demise, such as stillbirth (U.S. Department of Labor, n.d.). FMLA also extends leave to partners who are caring for their recovering spouse or partner. Although we know that the emotional scars often take longer to heal than the physical ones, you may be pressed to return to work for financial reasons or because of duties that require your presence. This pressure can add to your stress and feelings of despair. If you need more time off and you are in a position to do so, it is okay to ask for that time. You may need a note from your doctor, but it is important as part of your self-care to pay attention to your needs.

You may be hesitant to return to work because you are not yet ready to interact with people. Working from home, at least in the beginning, may be a good way to start if that is an option. Since the COVID-19 pandemic, many companies are more willing to be flexible in their requirements regarding in-person versus remote work.

However, this option is highly dependent on the type of work you do. Some jobs—such as flight attendant, medical practitioner, restaurant worker, or bank teller, to name a few—require the employee's physical presence. Perhaps you are self-employed and worried your business will collapse if you are absent for too long, or maybe you are a student and can't afford to miss class. Whatever your situation, you may want to inquire about whether you can ease back into full-time status if possible. Temporarily working part-time can give you a chance to test things out while still providing you more time to heal.

Malia: Challenges in the Workplace

Malia had a physically demanding job as a nurse in a local hospital emergency room. She needed to be on her feet for shifts that could last 12 hours, use her strength to position patients, assist patients with walking, carry equipment and supplies, and be ready for any emergency that occurred. Malia knew that it would be difficult to return to those demands full-time after her pregnancy loss, but she was also aware of the nursing shortage in her community. She was hesitant to approach her supervisor but realized it would be better to reduce the number of shifts she worked, at least for the near future. Her supervisor readily granted her request. Malia was in the fortunate position of working in a supportive and understanding environment at a job she truly loved.

As it happened, Malia was working one evening when a young woman came to the emergency room experiencing a miscarriage. At first, Malia panicked; she didn't want to work with this patient because it reminded her of her own loss. After Malia took a few deep breaths, however, she thought about what she needed during her loss and wanted to provide that for this patient. Her ability to help people through difficult life traumas was what drew her into the nursing field in the first place. Helping this woman in her pregnancy crisis was a way for Malia to heal as well.

What happens if you are not in a position like Malia's? Returning to a job that you do not enjoy, that is not fulfilling, or that is not accommodating can make it much worse. One complicating factor in returning to work is what coworkers know about your situation. Obviously, you have a right to privacy. But if people knew of your pregnancy, they will likely ask questions. What is the best way to communicate with them about your loss? Having an ally at the workplace, such as a supervisor or even a close coworker, can be a significant help. You can ask that person to let others know so you don't have to repeat your story to everyone you see when you return. There is nothing that says you must go into great detail; saying as much or as little as you want is fine.

Be prepared for awkward moments. Some coworkers may avoid you completely, which may make you feel self-conscious. Others may want to talk about your loss, even if you don't want to. These situations warrant digging into the toolbox again. If someone is avoiding you, you may have to approach them first to ease the awkwardness. On the other hand, if you don't want to discuss your loss with a coworker, you could simply say something like this: "Thank you for your concern, but I'm not ready to talk about it right now" or "Now is not a great time, but maybe we could have lunch together and talk?"

Even if you have an ally who can let others know your situation, it invariably happens that someone misses the memo or visits from another department and asks how the baby is. This situation can happen not only at work but also when you bump into someone who knew you were pregnant and assumes you had a baby. Depending on the relationship, you can go into detail or keep it simple. In these situations, often the person who congratulates you on having a baby feels utterly horrible and, in a reverse turn of events, you may wind up comforting them. When they apologize and say, "I'm so sorry, I had no idea," you may naturally want to soothe this uncomfortable interaction by telling them, "It's okay."

It is impossible to predict how returning to work will be for you. However, knowing ahead of time that there will likely be challenges—and having your toolbox at the ready—can help with this transition.

SUMMARY

I remember some sage advice I received from a clinical supervisor: "You can't stop bad things from happening, but you can learn to cope with disappointment and heartache." Your anguish can be overwhelming at times, especially in situations when you are dealing with people who don't understand pregnancy loss or say the wrong things. This chapter has suggested some practical ways to cope during those awkward times. Although the sting will still be there, with practice you will be able to get through it all and move forward.

Part of moving forward is the possibility of trying to conceive again. Chapter 7 focuses on how to navigate the emotional turmoil that can arise as you consider next steps and possibly different medical interventions. You have been through a trauma that can't be erased. You can, however, learn to cope with it, rewrite and edit your story, and manage your next steps.

CHAPTER 7

TRYING AGAIN: HOPE MIXED WITH A DOSE OF ANXIETY

Having a baby is commonly thought to be easy, yet it is a traumatic challenge for many. You, or someone close to you, has had a pregnancy loss—and perhaps more than one. If you are feeling anxious about trying to conceive again, you are not alone; nearly every person who has experienced a pregnancy loss lives with the dread that it will happen again. If you have a partner, they may also be afraid another pregnancy loss will occur, concerned about your well-being, and worried about the outcome. What will the next pregnancy be like? Will you be able to weather this together? How do you cope when every day—or perhaps every hour—feels like a roller coaster, with trepidation at one turn and hope at another? This chapter explores what it is like to become pregnant after a loss and provides strategies for managing anxiety as best you can.

FACING FEAR AND FINDING HOPE AFTER LOSS

Trying again after a pregnancy loss may prove to be treacherous emotionally. Not only are you grieving the baby who should have been, but you also now have a hefty dose of anxiety mixed with excitement over the possibility of another baby to come. Some people use the term *rainbow pregnancy* or *rainbow baby* to describe having a healthy baby after a pregnancy loss. The rainbow—a beautiful appearance after a storm—symbolizes hope after suffering through a painful, dark, and chaotic time. Regardless of the terminology used, think about all the emotions at play when considering this experience: sadness, hope, depression, elation, worry, excitement, fear—the list goes on and on. Trying again can be stressful; you likely have many questions regarding how best to move forward, and you may especially want to have control over the outcome. The following case of Dana illustrates the impact of a previous loss on a subsequent pregnancy. This case provides a glimpse into some of Dana's therapy sessions with me, followed by my commentary on the process. Through examining Dana's experience and following her in therapy, you will learn strategies to manage your own emotions.

DANA: UNRELENTING ANXIETY

Dana, a 34-year-old high school math teacher, was pregnant again 8 months after her first miscarriage. She was concerned that it had taken so long to get pregnant again, and now she was worried she would have another miscarriage. Now that Dana was pregnant, she said her anxiety was "through the roof!" She started therapy with me after a particularly difficult, angst-ridden morning.

Therapy Session 1

Dana: I can't tell you how many times I go to the bathroom to check: Is there blood, or am I still okay? I've been so scared. I haven't wanted to do anything—even go for a walk—because what if that causes me to bleed? And then on Monday morning, I really lost it, and that's when I knew I had to make an appointment. When I woke up, I thought I felt

> dampness in my underwear. And my breasts, which had felt so sore for the past 2 weeks, were only a little tender. Not like they had been, and not like they had been the first time I was pregnant. I sat up in bed and began to sob, and I couldn't stop. Geoff tried to soothe me; he actually went into the bathroom with me to check my underwear. When there was no blood, you would think I would calm down, but I started to hyperventilate, had sweaty palms, and thought I was going to pass out. I just couldn't catch my breath. Geoff was amazingly calm through the whole thing; he thought I was having a panic attack, and he just held me. We both agreed that if I was going to get through this pregnancy—no matter what the outcome—I was going to need some counseling. So here I am.

Dana's introduction came out in a rush. She was anxious about the pregnancy, exasperated by starting therapy, and fearful of being judged: What would I think of her? Would I understand? It was important for her to feel supported and to know that her reactions, although very upsetting, were not unexpected, and I acknowledged this in my reply.

> *Dr. J:* You are dealing with so much right now. Not only are you grieving the loss of your first pregnancy, but you are so afraid of losing this one as well. Of course you are feeling anxious. How could you feel any other way?

Dana took a deep breath. Although she had tears in her eyes, she started to relax.

Session 1 Commentary: Validation

As mentioned previously in this volume, you may have received unhelpful comments from others (e.g., "Just get over it" or "Don't dwell on it") after a pregnancy loss. Similarly, when you become pregnant again, the expectation is that you should feel nothing but joy. These optimistic sentiments don't come close to the complex emotions you experience—excitement and hope mixed with fear and dread. A first step in managing the storm of emotions thundering in your head and heart is to give them a voice in a safe and secure place. That place can be with family and friends, but they may be so emotionally wrapped up in protecting you that they may offer unwanted advice and want to fix it. This is where talking with a professional—be it a psychologist, social worker, counselor, or clergyperson—can be beneficial. Healing begins when you, with all your tumultuous and sometimes contradictory emotions, are truly heard. Letting Dana know that her anxiety was warranted given the situation was a way to validate and normalize her feelings.

Therapy Session 2

Dana: I've been trying to figure out what went wrong, what caused the miscarriage. My doctor told me that it wasn't my fault—that it was probably caused by a genetic anomaly. He said, "It's nature's way of ensuring a healthy baby," but I keep thinking about what I did. That I did something wrong.

Dr. J: [*Inquiring gently*] You don't believe what your doctor told you?

Dana: No, no, I do, but . . .

Dr. J: Tell me what you think you did to cause your loss.

Dana: I don't know. I had a glass of wine—it was before I knew I was pregnant. And I rearranged the desks in my classroom. Maybe I did too much.

Dr. J: [*Reassuringly*] Dana, I understand your concerns. I don't know anyone who has had a pregnancy loss who doesn't wonder if they somehow caused it. If you knew that you did something to cause it, of course you wouldn't do it again.

I gave Dana some examples of self-blame that women had shared with me.

Dr. J: One woman was convinced that she caused her miscarriage by getting a pedicure, thinking the nail polish fumes were to blame. Another woman thought it was the jelly beans she ate—and of course she never ate them again!

Dana smiled. It was helpful for her to hear she was not alone.

Dana: I guess I'm being silly.

Dr. J: No, I don't think it's silly at all. What you're looking for is some way to be in charge of this pregnancy. So much is going on inside your body right now that is out of your conscious control. Trusting that your body knows what to do to support this growing baby is hard.

Session 2 Commentary: Longing for Control

Self-blame is a common reaction to a pregnancy loss. Paradoxically, it can feel better to blame yourself than to not have something concrete to hold on to. Of course, if there were something you could do (or not do) to guarantee that this pregnancy would be successful, you would do it. If you recall our discussion of the fundamental assumptions that form the solid foundations that guide us through life (Chapter 3, this volume), you'll remember that control is one of the basics. Wanting to be in control of your subsequent pregnancy is the most natural desire, even if there really is not much you can do other than eat well, take your prenatal vitamins, get enough sleep and exercise, and go to your obstetric appointments—all the basics of prenatal self-care.

Although it may not feel like enough, it can be helpful to remind yourself that getting and staying pregnant is not a skill. In fact, pregnancy is a complex biochemical process that essentially runs on its own. Telling yourself this repeatedly, almost like a mantra, can help manage your anxiety. Unless you have an underlying medical condition that needs to be monitored, most routine activities will not cause your pregnancy to fail. Of course, if you are concerned about any of your activities, you should consult with your health care provider.

Therapy Session 3

Dana: I hear what you and my doctor are saying—I didn't cause the miscarriage to happen. But I have been so stressed about having another miscarriage, so stressed that something will go wrong with this pregnancy. I mean, isn't there evidence that too much stress is harmful?

Dr. J: Stress is a complicated phenomenon. Yes, in general, it can lead to some negative health effects, but it is so dependent on one's perception of the stressful experience and how well one responds to it, how much resiliency one has, and how one copes with it. There is no doubt that having a miscarriage is stressful. And I don't know anyone who has had a loss who is not anxious during a subsequent pregnancy. It's a normal response.

Dana: And how do you make sure that someone is stressed out? [*Chuckles*] Tell them to relax!

Dr. J: Exactly! The last thing we want is for you to feel like you're not relaxing enough. That would be like blaming the victim of a crime instead of the criminal. The fact that you are here seeking support says to me that you are taking some action to help yourself. That is an indicator of your coping skills. And that's what we will work on together—increasing your coping skills to decrease your stress.

Session 3 Commentary: Stress and Pregnancy

We know that infertility and pregnancy loss cause stress, and there have been numerous studies that support these findings (Bhat & Byatt, 2016; Galst, 2018; Rooney & Domar, 2018). However, there are also many questions regarding the reverse—that is, whether stress causes reproductive traumas to occur. To better understand the relationship between stress and pregnancy, it is helpful to review how perinatal loss was regarded historically and to examine how much this thinking has changed over time. Historically, early explanations of reproductive loss were explained by the *psychogenic theory*, which proposed that pregnancy losses and infertility were caused by unconscious conflicts women had about becoming a mother. Stated another way, women's mental stressors were thought to be the cause of reproductive problems. All negative reproductive issues were blamed on women (Leon, 1996).

Advances in reproductive medicine have now largely debunked the psychogenic theory. For example, we know that infertility affects men and women equally. Some estimates indicate that approximately one-third of infertility cases can be attributed to female factors, one-third to male factors, and one-third to both (American Society for Reproductive Medicine, 2023a). Greater medical knowledge of genetics and increased prenatal testing have also informed us of some of the physical issues that cause pregnancy loss.

Although the role that stress plays in pregnancy loss has evolved, stress may still interfere with your sense of well-being. Later in this chapter, several stress-reducing strategies are introduced. These interventions will not increase your chances of getting or staying pregnant, but they have been shown to reduce stress and overwhelming anxiety. Using these strategies will help you feel better and be able to manage and cope better, even if you are not able to control the pregnancy outcome.

Therapy Session 4

Aside from acknowledging Dana's emotional state, I wanted to understand what having a family meant to her. Her response would give me insight into her reproductive story and how the trauma of pregnancy loss had wreaked havoc on her beliefs about children and relationships in her family.

Dana: You know, no one has ever asked me about this—about what it means to me to have a family of my own. [*Pauses a moment to reflect*] I have a lot of friends who have decided they don't want to have kids because they are worried about the climate crisis and unstable political leaders around the world. But for me—and Geoff—I think we see having children as a beacon of light for the future. I see it in my students who are excited about learning. I don't know . . . being able to nurture and love a child . . . maybe it's selfish, but I can't imagine going through life without that experience. It's one thing to foster this in my students but quite another to mold a life with a child of my own.

Dana sat quietly for a moment with her hands clenched in her lap before she continued.

Dana: This might sound weird, but I want to have kids for my grandmother before she dies. She taught me so much about life; I want to pass that on. She would get such joy from this. I can see that photo in my mind—four generations posing together—that's family. [*Looks down and starts to cry*] I'm so afraid it's not going to happen. [*Pauses and looks up*] So how do I stop this constant worry? I can't spend every day in panic mode, waiting for the other shoe to drop! I'm just so scared I'll have another miscarriage!

Session 4 Commentary: Coping Strategies

As we have discussed, a pregnancy loss represents more than the baby-to-be. Dana listed her worries about not being able to experience parenthood. She also had a strong desire to maintain family traditions and feel a sense of continuity from one generation to the next. She felt responsible, with the weight on her shoulders to make sure this would happen. Her baby represented the future as well as the legacy of the past.

Reflecting on your own story and what creating a family means to you can be an important tool in understanding your anxiety, especially as you are trying to conceive again. You may be feeling a lot of pressure, as Dana did; and you may be worried that your chance to become a parent is slipping away. The anxiety of waiting is enormous. Whether it's waiting for a positive pregnancy test or waiting for the various gestational milestones throughout a pregnancy, the experience is nerve-wracking. Dana and I discussed ways she had coped with stressful situations in the past. Would it be possible for her to incorporate some of those strategies now? We also considered various other ways she might reduce her anxiety. These coping strategies are presented next for you to try as well.

BUILDING YOUR OWN COPING STRATEGIES

In addition to the emotional toolbox you've developed to cope with baby showers, holidays, birthdays, weddings, and other social events (Chapter 6, this volume), it is important to also have strategies to manage your own overwhelming feelings when you are trying again. As you read through these suggestions, some ideas may resonate more than others. You can pick and choose different strategies, try some out and come back to try others, and add what works to your emotional toolbox.

Say It Out Loud

Sitting with the overwhelming feelings and understanding your own backstory can be paradoxically soothing. Giving voice to your emotions by literally saying them out loud can reduce much of the sting. This was true for Dana in our earlier case example: After she reflected on what having a baby meant to her, the tension in her body dissipated. She unclenched her hands, her shoulders relaxed, and she took a deep breath.

One of the positive outcomes of telling your story repeatedly is that each time you tell it, you are in a different emotional place. You change with each telling; you grow from reflecting on your story. In our case example, Dana had never put into words the reasons this pregnancy meant so much to her. Gaining a better understanding of yourself is one of the hallmarks of psychotherapy.

Similarly, identifying your anxiety triggers allows you to manage them better. Dana was acutely aware of the bodily sensations of pregnancy. Her anxiety exploded when she was sure her body was telling her something was wrong. You too may be keenly aware of every pain, every bit of nausea, every headache, or every absence of typical pregnancy symptoms. The problem is that your interpretations may be faulty. Just because you felt nauseous yesterday but not today does not mean that something is wrong. Listening to yourself—feeling what you feel—won't necessarily erase the worry, but identifying what triggers your anxiety can help.

Write About Your Feelings

Keeping a journal is another productive way to give voice to your feelings. The beauty of journaling is that you can do it whenever you need to get something off your chest. Writing in your journal can act as a brain dump exercise, so to speak: You can feel and write anything you want, which you may be more hesitant to do with a live person listening. Journals can help to organize your thoughts and allow you to reflect. Looking back over past entries enables you to see how you have changed over time or how some issues continue to persist.

Some people balk at the idea of writing about their feelings. One woman said she didn't want anyone to read what she wrote.

It wasn't that she thought writing would be unhelpful; rather, it was so private that she didn't want to share it with anyone or have a record of her feelings. So after she finished writing, she made a ritual of shredding the paper. As she said, "It was like—poof—the feelings vanished into thin air."

Make a Plan

In one of our sessions, Dana described how she was overcome with anxiety in the middle of teaching a math class one day.

> I found myself suddenly overwhelmed. I have no idea what triggered it, but I was having a hard time concentrating on what I was trying to teach. All I could think about was running to the bathroom to check for blood. Obviously, I couldn't do that!

However, Dana could use the restroom between classes, regardless of whether nature was calling, and we made this her plan. "Am I being too obsessive about this? When am I going to trust that it's going to be okay?" she wondered. We agreed that, at least for now, knowing she had a plan in place helped to quell her anxiety.

Another strategy is to create *worry time* for yourself. This technique is used in cognitive behavior therapy, and it suggests you set aside a specific time every day to go over your worries. Depending on your needs, it can last from about 15 to 30 minutes. The idea is that rather than spend time on your anxieties as they percolate throughout the day, you set aside a specific time frame to focus on them. If your anxiety is triggered by something during the day, you can note it and revisit it during your worry time. Remind yourself that you will have plenty of time to examine the situation later. It is recommended that you are consistent with the time and place you choose (e.g., say, 8 p.m. every evening while sitting at your desk or kitchen table). As you focus during worry time on the things that have you stressed, think about whether you can find a solution to your worries.

It can also be helpful to make a note of what happened right before you felt overcome with anxiety and worry. Did you feel something physically? Did someone make a comment that upset you? Were you in a situation that made you uncomfortable? As noted earlier, Dana relied on her bodily sensations to assure herself that the pregnancy was going in the right direction. Because Dana knew she was susceptible to these feelings, being able to predict them allowed her to rein in some of the anxiety. Doctor's appointments are another time when anxiety can surface. The fear that there won't be a heartbeat or that the baby isn't growing as expected is heightened prior to checkups. By predicting when worries are more likely to occur, you can prepare yourself emotionally. The objective is to allow you to have more control over them.

Remember the Good

When you are experiencing loss and trauma, it can be hard to believe that anything good could come from it. In Chapter 8, we'll focus on the many ways we can grow from adversity and change. Researchers call this *posttraumatic growth* (PTG; Tedeschi et al., 2015; Triplett et al., 2012), and we can think of it as the silver lining that occurs with examination of the trauma and the positive way one's life can grow out of the negative situation. PTG does not occur immediately after a traumatic event; as you will see, it develops over time.

In the short term, there are ways to work on negative thoughts and feelings. *Positive reappraisal coping intervention* (PRCI) is one such technique. Psychological studies have noted the positive effects of utilizing PRCI with individuals who have experienced recurrent miscarriages and in the waiting period after intrauterine insemination (Bailey et al., 2015; Ghasemi et al., 2017). The idea behind this practice is that when you are feeling stressed or anxious, you can turn to messages you created for yourself—whether on your phone or a piece of paper—that remind you of other ways of thinking. The objective is to interrupt the negative spiral of your emotions by reviewing your list of reappraisals throughout the day. The research on PRCI suggests that you should include 10 items on your list (Bailey et al., 2015; Ghasemi et al., 2017). For example, we know that waiting to find out whether you are pregnant (i.e., what is commonly called the *2-week wait*) can produce a great deal of anxiety. An item on your PRCI list could say, "I know this is not going to last forever." You might also include a statement such as, "These are just feelings, they will go away" or "It's normal to feel this way given what I have gone through." Because Dana was so concerned about having another miscarriage, she misinterpreted every bodily shift as something going wrong. Included in her list was this positive statement: "Sensations are just sensations and not necessarily true, especially when I'm anxious." Dana added yet another affirmation to her list: "I'm afraid of having another miscarriage, but I got through the last one. And if it happens again, I know I'll get through it too." These are just some examples of what you can include in your list. In Exercise 7.1, I encourage you to reflect on your own situation and apply PRCI. What negative thoughts and feelings have you been dwelling on? Challenge yourself to write positive affirmations for each.

EXERCISE 7.1. Your Positive Reappraisals

List 10 situations that are upsetting you. For each item on your list, think about a positive coping statement that will help you get through it. You can write your positive reappraisals on an index card and put it in your pocket or purse, or you can store them on your phone. You want to carry your list around with you, so you can pull it out periodically during the day or whenever you feel your emotions taking over.

Practice Daily Gratitude

To-do lists can be wonderful ways to stay organized. They can help you prioritize the things you need to do, with the most important items high on the list. Checking off the things that you've accomplished can be so satisfying. If you are like most people, there may be more on your to-do list than you can reasonably achieve in a day; also, what likely stands out most are the things that didn't get done. If you are overcome with depression and anxiety, it can also be more difficult to feel that you have accomplished anything.

Instead of focusing on what you haven't achieved, take a moment to think about what you completed on your to-do list or what you appreciated during the day. They don't have to be big things. Maybe you made a phone call or answered an email. Maybe you did the laundry or went for a walk. Maybe you savored the cup of coffee you had this morning, or perhaps you appreciated a friend who reached out to say hello.

Perhaps it is human nature to focus on the negative, which is especially true when you are grieving and overwhelmed with anxiety if you are trying to conceive again. It may feel like a challenge to find gratitude in the small things that fill your day. Practicing *daily gratitude*, or consciously being thankful for something in your life, has been shown to enhance not only mental health but also physical health (Wise et al., 2012).

A good way to practice daily gratitude is to keep a journal and write down three things that you feel grateful for. Some people find it best to do this before bedtime when they can reflect on the day. Even if you don't keep a journal, just thinking about three things—giving yourself credit for what you achieved and what you are thankful for—is an important element of self-care, especially when you are hurting. Utilizing this kind of compassion for yourself is yet another component of healing.

Mindful Moments

Mindfulness is the practice of purposely paying attention to the moment you are in and staying present in that moment (Kabat-Zinn, 2021). Instead of ruminating about the past or fretting about the future, mindfulness is a conscious effort to be fully in the present. Mindfulness-based 8-week workshops and training programs that incorporate relaxation, breathing exercises, meditation, yoga, and cognitive behavior therapy have been shown to help reduce stress (Khoury et al., 2015). Taking a *mindful moment* when you are stressed has also been suggested as a way to reset your thoughts; this can act as a momentary escape from the anxiety you are feeling (Norcross & Phillips, 2020).

So how do you create mindful moments? A simple way to start is to sit quietly, close your eyes, and focus on your breathing. Your mind might wander, and that's okay. You can bring yourself back to the moment by just observing your breath—not changing it in any way but just observing it. Another way to create a mindful moment is to take the time to really look at something. Perhaps you look at a piece of artwork, examining the colors, shapes, and design. Or maybe you look at a flower, seeing its structure and smelling its fragrance. Yet another idea is to be mindful when you are doing a chore, such as washing the dishes. Instead of just getting through it, notice how the water feels on your hands. Is it warm? Is it cool? How does it feel running over your fingers? Listen for the sounds the water makes as it runs out of the faucet. Does the soap you use have a fragrance? Concentrate on the bubbles it makes. Can you see colors in the soap suds? Perhaps you can think lovingly about cleaning the pots and pans that provide the means for nourishment. Now notice how it feels to dry your hands. Is the towel soft? Can you slow down to give each finger equal attention in the drying process, maybe even massaging each one as you go?

Paying attention to these kinds of details, engaging as many of your senses as possible, allows you to focus and slow down. If you are feeling overwhelmed by anxiety, worried about attempting to get pregnant again, or feeling triggered by grief, taking a mindful moment can serve as a brief pause that allows your busy mind to rest. This can take just seconds to do, and you can do it anywhere, anytime, and whenever you feel like it throughout the day.

Exercise, Yoga, and Your Mental Health

If you are grieving and feeling depressed, the idea of doing any kind of exercise may be completely unappealing. Your body needs time to heal but so does your mind, and you may just not feel up to doing anything physical. This is totally understandable given the loss you have experienced. While you may just feel like crawling under the covers and mindlessly watching a video (a practice that does have its benefits for tuning out the world), the evidence for bolstering mental health through exercise is abundant. Studies suggest that exercise not only improves physical well-being, but it also has a positive effect on mood and decreases anxiety (Smith & Merwin, 2021).

Exercise has also been shown to have positive benefits during pregnancy. Not only does exercise help control excessive gestational weight gain and blood pressure, but it is also associated with a higher incidence of vaginal births and lower rates of cesarean delivery (American College of Obstetricians and Gynecologists Committee on Obstetric Practice, 2020). Here is a note of caution: Before you engage in any form of exercise prior to getting pregnant or during pregnancy, consult with your doctor. The recommendations suggested here are general and not specific to you or your situation. You may be hesitant to do anything physical when trying again, for fear that you would cause another loss. Not surprisingly, this is the reason women often give when they mention not wanting to exercise, even though the benefits of regular exercise and its safety have been noted throughout the research (American College of Obstetricians and Gynecologists, 2022; Berghella & Saccone, 2017).

What exercises should you avoid? Sports such as horseback riding, downhill skiing, water skiing, surfing, gymnastics, or any activity that presents a fall risk should be avoided. Likewise, it is advisable to steer clear of activities where you might be hit or kicked, such as boxing, ice hockey, basketball, soccer, or judo. Scuba diving and skydiving can increase your risk of injury. Safe exercises during pregnancy include walking, swimming, or stationary cycling.

Yoga, modified for pregnancy, is another recommended form of exercise. Yoga consists of stretching and strength building poses (*asanas*), along with breathing and meditation. Because yoga practice combines movement with relaxation, it is beneficial for women who are trying to conceive or are pregnant after a loss. The physical advantages of yoga are numerous, including controlled stretching of skeletal muscles, adding strength and balance. The psychological benefits of yoga are also valuable: The asanas, combined with self-reflection, concentration, and relaxation, can reduce the overriding emotions of anxiety, sadness, and depression that plague women after a loss and when they are trying again.

Many styles of yoga are practiced, although some should be avoided during pregnancy. For example, hot yoga during pregnancy is not recommended because it can potentially increase your body temperature to dangerous levels. As with all forms of exercise during pregnancy, again remember this critical point: Check with your health care provider before engaging in any yoga practice. Then find a yoga instructor who is well versed in pregnancy, because some poses must be modified to accommodate your changing body. For example, you may not want to do asanas that put pressure on your abdomen; with a trained prenatal yoga provider, the asanas can be customized to fit your needs.

WHEN TO SEE YOUR DOCTOR

Think back to Dana, whose anxiety about being pregnant again was difficult to control. She desperately wanted to be reassured that her current pregnancy would not suffer the same fate as the previous one. "I went in for an appointment this week," Dana began. "Everything is looking good. I felt relieved, of course. But the relief lasted about a day and then the anxiety started up again. The wait between appointments is so long," she cried.

The need for assurance is common in subsequent pregnancies. "I have had other clients who have felt exactly the same way," I said, validating Dana's feelings. I suggested the following:

> You might want to talk with your clinic and see if you can come in more frequently. I've known other women who have done this. They were surprised that their doctors were so accommodating, but a quick check of the baby's heartbeat made them feel so much better. It might be worth asking if that's possible.

Some women experiencing pregnancy-related anxiety decide to rent or buy a fetal Doppler ultrasound monitor. The Doppler allows you to hear your baby's heartbeat, but it does not have imaging capability. It may seem like a no-brainer to get one; after all, if it helps you feel more secure and know that your pregnancy is progressing, why not? I have known women who have sworn by the Doppler, while others decided it would probably cause more anxiety rather than less. It is sometimes difficult to find a baby's heartbeat with the Doppler, even for trained technicians: This doesn't mean something is wrong. The baby simply may be in a position that makes it harder to find the heartbeat, yet this scenario still increases your anxiety. The Doppler can also give a false sense of security if it picks up your heartbeat instead of the baby's.

If only you had a window into the mysterious growth and development of your child. In early pregnancy, it can feel unsettling when the only indicators you have are your own nausea and fatigue. As your pregnancy progresses, you may be reassured by feeling fetal movement. Even then, subsequent pregnancies can feel like a long waiting game until your baby is born. It is very difficult to trust the process, especially if you have had a previous loss. The bottom line is this: If at any point you think that something is wrong, it is best to see your doctor.

DOES A SUBSEQUENT PREGNANCY MAKE THE HURT GO AWAY?

It goes without saying that your loss is like no other. When there is death where there should have been life, there are no words to describe this devastation. You may feel as if the only way to heal from your loss is to try to have another child as soon as possible. In fact, people may have told you that "you'll feel better when you have a baby"; although they mean well, having another baby doesn't make all the hurt go away. You cannot simply replace your baby (or hoped-for baby) with another; what you may want is for that baby, that pregnancy, to be progressing as you had hoped.

Both women and men feel intensified anxiety with a subsequent pregnancy. It is hard not to compare the new pregnancy with the previous one. Women carry the pregnancy and thus may be hypervigilant, waiting for something to go wrong. Sometimes, in an effort to ward off the pain of another demise, a woman may try not to attach to the current fetus. Even if that were possible, it doesn't guarantee that the feelings of grief and loss would be any less strong. Guilt can also play a powerful role, with the woman feeling as if she is abandoning the previous baby for the current one. Knowing that her heart—and love—can extend to both is helpful. It is not necessary to reject one baby to be loyal to the other. Likewise, one can grieve the past and embrace the future at the same time. For men, there is a tendency to put their own needs aside to protect their partner through the subsequent pregnancy. Although their grief and anxiety may be just as intense, they may try to hide their feelings to appear strong and supportive. They may feel on guard, keeping a watchful eye over their partner's health and well-being.

A subsequent pregnancy won't take all the pain away. However, a successful pregnancy and birth can bring some resolution. Knowing that your body can get pregnant and carry to term can be healing. It can also be fulfilling to finally get to join with and identify with other parents, especially as a first-time parent. Having a baby after going through a loss is complicated, with many opposing feelings occurring at the same time. Joy and grief, as well as excitement and anxiety, all mixed with love are normal reactions to having a baby after a loss.

WHAT IF IT'S ALL TOO MUCH? GIVING YOURSELF PERMISSION TO STOP

Although this chapter focuses on trying again after a loss, sometimes it can feel like it's just too hard. The emotional toll is overwhelming; the possibility of going through another loss can be so overpowering that you just don't want to go down that road again. One woman described walking into her doctor's office again this way:

> The fluorescent lights, the medical smell of the place, the staff in their white coats—it felt like I was in an episode of the *Twilight Zone*. I had to get out of there. It became clear that I needed to rethink what I wanted for the future.

Another woman was told that to get pregnant, she would need surgery to remove scar tissue in her uterus. She shared, "They told me that there's no guarantee, and I could still have a miscarriage. Do I really want to take that risk?"

Think back to your original reproductive story. How far afield has it gone? Have your goals changed? What possibilities await you in the future? If your goals include having children, there are many paths you can follow to achieve that goal, as discussed thoroughly in Chapter 9. Perhaps your reproductive story is evolving in other, unexpected ways. If you already have a child or children, you may decide that your current family is fine the way it is and doesn't need to grow. If you don't have children, you may choose to focus your energy in a different direction; this will be discussed in Chapter 8, when we learn about PTG.

It is important to remember that you have choices. You may not have been able to control all the events that have led you here, but you can make decisions about your future—whether you decide to pursue the journey to parenthood or a different journey. Life has changed from the way you thought it would be, but being open to the new possibilities ahead can lead you to places unimagined before.

SUMMARY

The stakes are high when you attempt to get pregnant again. The worry and angst that you may feel is normal and to be expected given what you have experienced. The good news is that, for many people, the odds of conceiving again and having a healthy baby are still in your favor, whether you suffered a miscarriage, stillbirth, ectopic pregnancy, or other perinatal loss.

Getting through a subsequent pregnancy is emotionally challenging. This chapter focused on a variety of coping strategies—some may feel right for you, and others may not. The goal is to try different ideas to help you manage your grief, anxiety, and depression and see what fits. Remember that reducing your stress will not help with conception, but it may make you feel better about yourself, your relationships, and life in general.

This chapter discussed ways of dealing with stress and anxiety in the immediacy of your loss and a possible subsequent pregnancy. In the next chapter, we'll focus on how people can change and grow from adversity in the long term, which is referred to as *posttraumatic growth*. Although it may not seem possible that anything positive could arise from reproductive trauma, we'll examine the positive ways one's life can evolve after these negative events.

CHAPTER 8

FROM REPRODUCTIVE TRAUMA TO GROWTH: HEALING AND CHANGE

Most of us are aware of the phenomenon of posttraumatic stress disorder (PTSD). As discussed in Chapter 3 (this volume), a reaction to a traumatic event can trigger any or all of the following symptoms: intense anxiety or depression (or both), flashbacks or an intrusive reliving of the event, sleep disturbances, and feelings of agitation or numbness (American Psychiatric Association, 2022). In Chapter 3, we noted that many people who experience reproductive loss have these symptoms and may receive a diagnosis of PTSD. Even if your symptoms do not fit the full criteria of a PTSD diagnosis, you may still be traumatized by your pregnancy loss. As we discussed, grieving, processing the loss, and learning how to cope with it are all ways to help you heal from the devastation of your reproductive dreams being shattered.

A new focus of research is *posttraumatic growth* or PTG (Tedeschi et al., 2015; Triplett et al., 2012). Although the concept of PTG is as old as time—that is, out of adversity, growth will occur—formal research into the phenomenon, especially as it relates to disruptions of the reproductive story, is relatively new. Some studies have examined PTG and infertility (Ayalti & Bayraktar, 2017; Paul et al., 2010; Yu et al., 2014; Zhang et al., 2021), others have assessed PTG and pregnancy loss (Alvarez-Calle & Chaves, 2023; Krosch &

Shakespeare-Finch, 2017; Ryninks et al., 2022; Winograd, 2017), and yet other research has focused on PTG and parental bereavement (Waugh et al., 2018). The results of these studies all point to the same conclusion: PTG was identified regardless of the type of loss suffered, and it was seen across individuals in a variety of cultures and ethnicities.

In previous chapters, we concentrated on the steps you can take to practice coping in moments of grief and loss, with the aim to help you get by in the immediate aftermath of your loss (Chapter 6) and to help you cope with trying again (Chapter 7). With its focus on PTG, this chapter will introduce you to the silver lining of possibilities that can occur as a result of a tragic pregnancy loss. One thing to keep in mind is that PTG does not erase the experience of the loss; you have been forever transformed by it. PTG does, however, open avenues in your life—both big and small—that address how you have been changed by the trauma. Reproductive losses are indeed life-altering events. To grow from them, it is important to understand how you have been affected and changed by your loss; its impact on you, your relationships, and your life is at the heart of this chapter.

PTG develops over time: You will not experience it immediately after your loss; your perspective will change and grow over months and years. Readers of this book are at different stages in their grief and loss. You may not yet be able to fully grasp any changes that may have occurred in your perspective of the world. The assumptions you had have been shattered, and it takes time to evaluate and construct new outlooks on life. Therefore, I recommend you read this chapter now but understand that you should come back to it and reread it later. It might be helpful to keep a record of your responses to and thoughts about the ideas presented here, and then review them after some time has passed—say, 6 months, a year, or 2 years. In doing so, you will be able to note how your attitude and perceptions of yourself have changed, and you will be able to measure how your reproductive trauma has opened avenues of growth.

REBUILDING FROM REPRODUCTIVE TRAUMA

Think back to the core assumptions we discussed in Chapter 3. These include benevolence, predictability, and control, which are defined as follows:

- *Benevolence* is the idea that kind and caring people fill your world. This assumption allows you to trust in other people and have confidence in yourself.
- *Predictability* is the assumption that your life has structure and that you can and do make plans for yourself. It allows you to know what to expect. There is comfort in that.
- *Control* describes your ability to set into motion the plans you have made and see them through to the finish line.

These three assumptions are the structural foundations of our belief systems, the solid ground on which we base our lives, and the building blocks of solid relationships. Our hopes and dreams are based on these beliefs; when they are thrown into disarray, nothing feels right. The world as we knew it and as we believed in it has been upended. When a reproductive trauma occurs, the solid foundation that we have counted on is shattered into pieces.

Think about a house that has been built on these assumptions. The construction of the house is solid, and you anticipate that you will live in the house—and make it your home—for many years to come. But what happens if a devastating earthquake, fire, or flood occurs? Your house has been damaged, and you need to take stock of the destruction. What needs to be replaced? What can be salvaged out of the ruins? Before you can really grasp the totality of what has happened and how to rebuild, you need to examine and reflect on the damages. You need to understand the impact this loss has had on your life.

The same kind of cognitive reappraisal takes place when a negative reproductive event occurs. Your assumptions of creating a family have been shattered. As you take stock of the damage to your sense of self, your relationships with others, and your dreams, you may not believe that you will be able to rebuild your life, but you will. A new worldview can come into being out of the trauma. It is the cognitive rebuilding of your shattered assumptions—the deep understanding of yourself and what has occurred—that allows for growth. Researchers have suggested that it is not the traumatic event itself that leads to PTG; rather, it is the struggle—the rebuilding—that occurs in the aftermath of the event that allows us to make sense of it (Ramos & Leal, 2013).

CONSTRUCTION, DECONSTRUCTION, AND RECONSTRUCTION

To gain further clarity, let's extend the house metaphor to the reproductive story. As we discussed in Chapter 2, the construction of your story began in your early childhood, with attention to play and mirroring of your vision of the adult world. In the building phase, you may have done some remodeling or made additions to your story as you went from being a child, through adolescence, then into adulthood. That is normal and to be expected. What is not expected is the destruction of your story—the circumstances surrounding the collapse of the house. Pregnancy loss and any disruption of the path to parenthood, including infertility and postpartum events, can bulldoze your expectations and change your life so deeply that you may not believe you can go on.

The reconstruction—the rebuilding—of your story, your life, and how and if you tackle another pregnancy is the focus of PTG. The reconstruction phase is the most important in terms of healing, growth, and the development of your future. When there is a discrepancy between your expectations and general beliefs of how pregnancy and parenthood should occur, it is natural to want to reduce this difference. This can be achieved by the work of grieving, understanding your pain, and finding new meaning for yourself. From the rubble of your previous assumptions of creating a family, you can reconstruct your ideas about what you want in your life and how to get there—whether that includes children or not. Figure 8.1 illustrates this process of construction, deconstruction, and reconstruction. It is important to remember that PTG is not a substitute for processing your grief and pain, but grief and PTG can and do coexist. While you are struggling to cope with your loss, positive change can occur at the same time.

FIGURE 8.1. The Path From Constructing to Rebuilding Your Reproductive Story

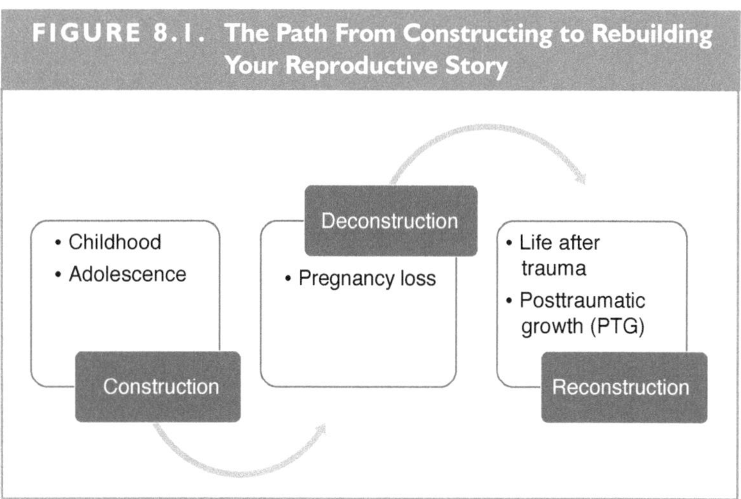

HOW DOES POSTTRAUMATIC GROWTH OCCUR?

Research points to three main elements needed for PTG to occur: (1) cognitive processing, (2) social support, and (3) self-disclosure (Tedeschi & Calhoun, 2004). Next, we'll dive into each of these areas and try to understand them in terms of reproductive loss.

Cognitive Processing

The research on PTG examines the thought processes that occur with trauma and loss (Triplett et al., 2012). To grow from the negative experience, you need to relive it, reexamine it, and reflect on how it has changed your life. At first, this may seem counterintuitive: Why would we want to reexperience the trauma in any way? Wouldn't it be best to block it out of our minds to move forward? The answer to these questions is no: Deliberate rumination on the loss helps us manage it and grow.

Two types of cognitive processing can occur. The first is *intrusive rumination*, which happens when thoughts or images occur automatically without your ability to control them. That is, they happen without you wanting them to, and you may feel as if you can't stop yourself from thinking about them. Perhaps you are triggered by something that causes a flashback to an unpleasant scene in the hospital. You may be flooded with emotion when you see someone else's newborn child. Or perhaps you are at a doctor's appointment when you suddenly feel lightheaded and overwhelmed with memories of seeing blood from a miscarriage. These types of thoughts are disturbing and can interfere with your well-being, leading to depression and increased anxiety. Intrusive thoughts do not help promote PTG. They can generate a great deal of distress, especially if they continue over a long period (Triplett et al., 2012).

In contrast, *deliberate rumination* is one key element that enables PTG to occur (Tedeschi & Calhoun, 2004). Deliberate rumination, as its name implies, is the process of intentionally thinking about the traumatic event. Rather than having thoughts randomly intrude, thinking about the trauma in a conscious, purposeful manner allows you to thoughtfully work through the experience. In essence, deliberate rumination is a way of making sense of the traumatic events. This kind of contemplation is a necessary step in understanding what happened and how it has changed your life. Whatever traumatic pregnancy loss you have endured, deliberate rumination allows you to put it into a context within your reproductive story and your life. You are in control of your thoughts, rather than your thoughts having control of you.

An effective way to ruminate deliberately may be to journal or write down your thoughts and feelings. Likewise, talking about the trauma can also help. Individual psychotherapy, peer group support, or couples therapy are all ways to process and share your thinking with others. Talking about it—with clergy, trusted friends, or family—may help you keep your anxiety in check. Deliberate contemplation can help to restore meaning and understanding to the disorder and disarray caused by the traumatic event. Thinking about it, writing about it, and sharing your thoughts with others are ways of making sense out of the chaos you have lived through. These strategies help in the rebuilding of your world and what it means for your future by incorporating this shift in your reproductive story.

Social Support

Social support is not the same as socializing with friends and family, although friends and family often offer social support. In general, *social support* can be defined as providing care and comfort, especially when someone is in a difficult situation. It can take the form of any number of acts of kindness, such as listening, providing food, or helping with chores. It can mean helping you get to your next doctor's appointment, being available to hold you when you feel like crying, or understanding how angry and upset you are. Social support is also about sharing information with others who are in a similar situation; finding other people who get it can provide a sense of belonging.

This kind of support takes two parties—one willing to give, and the other willing to receive. After a pregnancy loss, your knee-jerk reaction might be to isolate yourself. As much as isolation may seem helpful in the moment, it can be damaging in the long run. We know that isolation tends to lead to more isolation, which has been shown to increase depression and worsen physical health (Sherman et al., 2024). It is important to distinguish social support from social interactions. Social interactions, where you might be exposed to other pregnant people or babies, are not necessarily supportive, and you may feel the need to avoid them. However, connecting with trusted people who are there for you will help promote healing and growth.

Aside from family and friends, seeking professional help can feel like you have been thrown a life preserver in the middle of a tempest. Along with individual therapy, group therapy can be a great option. Groups can be led by professionals or peers, and they can be held in person or virtually. The benefits of talking with people who have experienced a similar loss are enormous. You can share information about medical issues, learn how others are coping, and know you are not alone. Many people I have worked with in therapy have found online support groups to be helpful in reducing their sense of isolation and shame. A support group may not be your preference, and that is perfectly fine; they are not for everyone. The main point is that seeking and receiving support—however feels right for you—is another important factor in the development of PTG.

Self-Disclosure

There is so much shame attached to pregnancy loss, as if one's self-worth is solely defined by having a child. Many highly successful and respected people lose all sense of their confidence when they experience infertility or pregnancy loss. Shame is one cause of isolation; it's that feeling of worthlessness that you have been unable to do what everyone else can—the seemingly simple task of having a baby. Add to that the guilt that percolates, as if you have done something wrong to cause your loss. Because reproductive losses are often discussed in hushed tones or not spoken about at all, it can feel as though you have done something improper, you have been cursed, and you need to bury your grief and loss.

Telling your story—sharing it repeatedly with trusted people in a supportive and safe environment—is a way to decrease your sense of shame. Giving voice to the darkest moments of your experience somehow lightens the load. It reduces feelings of isolation and self-blame. Talking about your story helps to make sense out of the unimaginable; this is part of the process of deliberate rumination. Not only can you begin to understand the loss better, but also you may see it slightly differently each time you disclose what you've been through. Exercise 8.1 can help with this process. Over time, this self-disclosure promotes PTG.

EXERCISE 8.1. The Upward Spiral of Growth

Think about a spiral that is elongated and has been stretched out—it has the shape of a tornado twisting from a central point upward. Imagine that you are starting at the bottom of the spiral but are moving upward along the trajectory. As you follow this path, sometimes it dips but the general direction is up. Each time you tell your story, you are moving along this route; at times there are downturns, but the spiral continues to rise. Each step along the way—each retelling—allows you to view and understand your loss in a slightly different way than before. Can you identify where you are right now on the spiral? Are you able to see where you started? How have you grown from that point?

HEALING TAKES TIME

No doubt you have heard the phrase "Time heals all wounds." If it were only that easy: All you would have to do is wait, and any and all hurt would simply go away. Here is another way to think about it: Healing, whether physically or mentally, takes time. Anyone who has fallen and scraped a knee or elbow knows that a scab will form, and you can watch as it gets smaller and heals. A bruise may turn black and blue at first but then slowly fade to other, softer shades over time before it eventually vanishes.

A central component to PTG is the amount of time since the trauma has occurred. Time allows you to gain perspective and think about yourself and the trauma differently. Immediately after a loss, you are in a state of crisis and shock. Processing the trauma and the shift in your reproductive story over time is necessary for growth to occur. In a study conducted with mothers whose child had died, researchers found that those who experienced the tragedy more recently reported less PTG than those who were further away from the trauma (Krosch & Shakespeare-Finch, 2017; Waugh et al., 2018). The time since the death was significantly correlated with levels of PTG.

The findings of Krosch and Shakespeare-Finch (2017) and Waugh et al. (2018) make intuitive sense. It takes time to heal. Just as the physical body needs time, rest, and medical care to recover from an injury, so does the emotional part of the self. While some injuries may vanish, others (e.g., a surgical scar) may be visible throughout one's life; this is also true for the emotional scars that remain after a pregnancy loss. It can be a lifelong process to make meaning and sense out of a reproductive trauma. Whatever your reproductive loss and struggle, you have been forever changed. As we will see in the following sections, the changes that occur in yourself are not all necessarily for the worse. Positive aspects of growth can and do occur over time as you heal.

One thing should be noted about the notion of time. Some early research on perinatal loss suggested that there is a *hierarchy of sadness* (Goldbach et al., 1991), which considered that the gestational age of the fetus determined the degree of loss. In other words, it was thought that the earlier the loss, the less pain was experienced. It would follow, then, that the less impact the loss has on you, the less chance for PTG. If you had an early miscarriage, you may have heard someone say, "Well, at least it happened early," as if that would make it easier to bear. These words are usually said to comfort, but they miss the mark. We know that the hierarchy of sadness is not true. Whether you have had an early miscarriage or have experienced a full-term stillbirth, it is not the gestational age of the pregnancy that matters; rather, it is the attachment you have to your pregnancy and to your baby, and what it means to you, that predicts grief and consequently the possibility of PTG (Lovell, 2001).

MEASURING GROWTH

How can you tell if you have grown from your reproductive loss? As noted earlier, you may not be able to recognize positive changes in yourself until some time has passed. Although the growth that emerges after a trauma can be seen as positive, that does not mean you must experience a traumatic event to grow. Growth can happen as life continues to unfold. However, the trauma can jolt your assumptions about life; it's almost like getting an electric shock, increasing your awareness of yourself, your surroundings, and your life. The silver lining to the massive disorder a traumatic experience creates is that personal growth and a new vision of life can blossom in its aftermath.

Researchers suggested that there are five distinct areas of growth (Figure 8.2):

- Gaining a greater sense of personal strength and competence
- Experiencing more intimate connections with others
- Having greater appreciation of life
- Questioning and/or developing spiritual beliefs
- Allowing for new pursuits and possibilities in your life (Ramos & Leal, 2013; Tedeschi et al., 2015)

These areas can be measured with the Posttraumatic Growth Inventory, the research tool most widely used to study PTG (Ramos & Leal, 2013; Tedeschi et al., 2015). Each area will be described next.

FIGURE 8.2. Five Areas of Growth

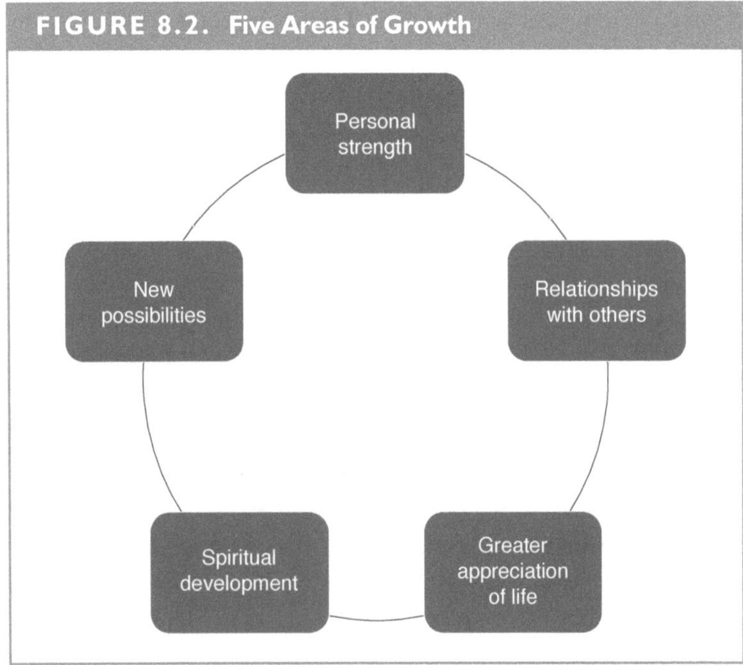

As you read through this section, think about yourself and the ways in which you have changed since your loss. As mentioned earlier, it would be helpful to note your responses and thoughts now and then to reexamine your reactions after some time has passed. Doing so will allow you to see how you have changed and grown over time.

Personal Strength

Think about a situation in your life that has been challenging—something that you have had to work hard at. Maybe it's studying to pass an exam, prepping for an important interview, or working under a deadline to get a project up and running. The feeling of accomplishment when you have successfully completed your goal fills you with a sense of pride and mastery. You did it! This is something that is within your control. That sense of competence in yourself grows with each daunting trial, building self-confidence.

These trials, however, pale in comparison to traumas that can occur in life—the events and situations that are not within your control. Traumatic experiences present the most challenging circumstances of all, with infertility and pregnancy loss ranking high among them. Living through these experiences can change your self-perception in a positive way. Although it may be hard to imagine how a pregnancy loss could possibly be positive, growth can occur. In dealing with this painful trauma, you become more in touch with your own feelings. Working through the hardships of a reproductive loss changes the way you see yourself. Yes, there is pain; but there is also a growing sense of self-confidence and power, knowing that you can move through it and move forward. The process of coping with pregnancy loss can transform you from feeling like a victim to becoming a survivor. This personal strength, assurance, and resiliency can be generalized to other situations in your life as well, with a belief that "if I can get through this, I can get through anything." Research has shown that people affected by a traumatic experience may feel more able to handle life's adversities and may feel a greater sense of inner strength than they thought they had (Tedeschi et al., 2015). Although no one would choose to experience a reproductive trauma, working through it can generate an inner sense of strength.

Relationships With Others

Not only is there a change in self-perception after trauma, but there is also a changed understanding of your relationships with other people. Think about the people who have been the most supportive to you during this time. You may feel closer to them than ever and appreciate them on a deeper level. Reproductive loss intensifies the preciousness of life, with a greater appreciation of those you care about deeply. Because of the continuing need to process and discuss your loss, you may be sharing more about yourself, and your willingness to accept support from others may be growing as well.

Relationships can also change in other ways. Sometimes it is only in the aftermath of a crisis that you discover who you can really count on. Some individuals you thought would provide support may be unable to, whereas other relationships may, in fact, grow stronger. This was true for Cynthia and her relationship with a close friend, Beth. The disruption caused by Cynthia's miscarriage seemed to shake not just her own world but also Beth's. Beth uncharacteristically ignored Cynthia's calls and texts after learning the news of Cynthia's pregnancy loss. Cynthia persisted and tried to understand why Beth was snubbing her. The answer became clear when Beth posted on social media that she was pregnant. Cynthia's hurt and anger grew. Why couldn't Beth be honest with her? It seemed Cynthia's loss was so frightening to newly pregnant Beth that she felt she needed to distance herself. Cynthia questioned the friendship, saw it in a different light, and realized that the rift might be too great to repair. However, another woman in their social group—aware of the negative dynamics that were interfering with their network of friends—reached out to Cynthia and extended more support, thus deepening their bond.

Growth can also occur with greater compassion for other people in general and especially for those who have been traumatized. If someone you know has experienced a similar reproductive traumatic event, your empathy for them may be more profound. For some, it may be only after their own pregnancy loss that they can more fully understand—and want to help—someone else in a similar position. One woman said, "It was only after I had a miscarriage that I understood what my friend had gone through. I feel terrible that I might have said the wrong things in trying to support her. My eyes are open now."

Learning about oneself through traumatic pregnancy experiences instills greater understanding and compassion for others. Often there is a desire to give back and want to help others going through a similar experience. As we will discuss in this chapter, this desire to help others is a prime example of PTG: It is sharing what you have learned from your own experience so that another person can be helped through theirs. Letting someone else know that they are not alone provides care and support.

Greater Appreciation of Life

One of the side benefits that PTG research has noted is a growing gratitude for the many small things that are part of life (Tedeschi et al., 2015). So often in our busy day-to-day routines, we may undervalue the little things that can fill us with pleasure. We may also take the people in our lives for granted, assuming and counting on their constant presence. Following trauma, research has noted that the people, the possessions we have, and the numerous ways life is filled with joy become more pronounced and are more valued (Tedeschi et al., 2015). Priorities and perspectives change. We don't take for granted even the smallest pleasures, and we can find ourselves appreciating these little treasures even more. Taking note of every time you smile or laugh during each day increases gratitude.

Consider this example of PTG. A patient came in with news that she needed to replace her refrigerator, which was an unexpected expense and annoyance.

> I opened the refrigerator to get out some milk for breakfast, but it wasn't at all cold. Then I opened the freezer, and all that food was soft and melting. I was able to salvage some stuff, but most of it had to be tossed. Of course it's upsetting, but it's not the end of the world. It's a hassle, but that's all it is. These things just don't get to me like they used to. At least the dishwasher is working!

Like many individuals, this patient had experienced a marked change in her philosophy of life, with a newfound perspective on the many trials and tribulations she faced. Things that would have been upsetting in the past take a backseat to what is really important in life.

Is it possible that the greater-appreciation-of-life aspect of PTG can affect one's subsequent role as a parent? Indeed, some research has found that previous reproductive trauma can positively affect subsequent parent–child relationships (Imrie & Golombok, 2018). For example, parents who struggled with infertility and opted to use egg donation to grow their family had more positive relationships with their children, with greater emotional involvement, compared with families who conceived naturally. They were also found to experience more joy in parenting (Imrie & Golombok, 2018). Some people who have struggled to have children (whether because of infertility, pregnancy loss, or both) may feel they don't have the right to complain about parenthood; they also may not take parenthood or their child or children for granted. Becoming a parent after traumatic loss can increase one's empathy for others, especially for one's children.

Spiritual Development

When a traumatic event occurs, deep questions can be raised. Here are some examples:

- Why did this happen to us?
- Am I being punished for something I did wrong?
- What is the point of my life if I can't have children?

These types of questions were haunting Alberto in the days and weeks after his wife, Gloria, was rushed to the hospital. They had been having dinner, discussing things they needed to set up a nursery. When Gloria got up to clear the table, her water broke. She was only 32 weeks pregnant, and the amniotic fluid–filled sac surrounding the baby had ruptured prematurely (known as *preterm premature rupture of membranes*). Gloria was put on bedrest in the hospital in an effort to maintain the pregnancy longer, but their son, Malcolm, was born 2 days later. He weighed only 3 pounds and lived in the hospital neonatal intensive unit for 10 days, but he did not survive. During the seemingly endless hours of watching Malcolm struggle to live, Alberto was wracked with questions about the meaning of life.

Everyone's spiritual beliefs are deeply personal. Some hold deep religious beliefs, while others may not. For some people, their faith can be strengthened by the trauma and loss; they may find great solace and strength in their religious beliefs and community. For others, the tragedy may weaken their beliefs and may foster more cynicism. It is not uncommon to question whether a just God would cause people to suffer.

Whether you are deeply religious, an atheist, or agnostic, your thoughts about yourself and your life have been challenged by reproductive loss. Regardless of your beliefs, whether they have been reinforced or diminished by the loss, you may find yourself thinking deeply about the meaning of life. This process of thinking about existential questions prompts PTG. As the research notes, the trauma can act as a trigger to search for new meaning and to find new pathways to achieve your goals (Tedeschi et al., 2015). Trying to make sense of it all is the catalyst for deeper awareness and growth, and perhaps discovering in yourself what you hold most dear. A new philosophy of life can emerge in the aftermath of reproductive trauma. Your perceptions of yourself, your relationships, and what is truly important in your life can change and develop in new and profound ways because of your loss.

New Possibilities

PTG may open new possibilities for you, ones that you may have never thought possible before. New ways to envision your life moving forward, and developing new plans and ambitions, are positive outcomes of trauma and loss. Discovering other aspects of yourself, making new choices, and creating new goals enable you to grow in unforeseen ways. The lessons people learn from traumatic experiences can, in the long run, create radical changes in how they live their life. As mentioned previously, the feeling of strength and mastery over the trauma ("If I can get through this, I can get through anything") allows you to try on different possibilities.

Sometimes the new avenues that people pursue develop directly out of the trauma they have endured. We see examples of this all the time. The parents of children who were victims of gun violence may become activists for gun reform. Survivors of sexual abuse often work with others to help them through the trauma. One young woman I know decided to study medicine after her mother died from breast cancer. The healing that can occur through taking action—going from a sense of helplessness to strength—cannot be overstated. Helping others through an experience that you have been through not only builds empathy but also opens new possibilities for yourself and your life. As we will discuss, many people who have suffered from reproductive trauma use their own loss to help others. As one patient said, "It's a way for me to give back after all the help and support I got."

There are many other ways that people explore new possibilities for themselves after trauma. Sometimes the trauma acts as the impetus to leave a job that has been unsatisfying. It can also inspire you to return to school or join in an activity that has been on your radar but you have been putting off. The question that prompts trying something new is this: "What is it that I really want?" While it is certainly possible to pursue new avenues in your life without trauma, the reflection on yourself, because of your traumatic experience, can be the catalyst for new pursuits.

As you reflect on new possibilities for yourself, you may discover different ways to envision your family. Think back to your reproductive story. That narrative—emerging from childhood through imagining what becoming a parent would be like—has been thwarted by the reproductive trauma that you have experienced. You have had to rewrite your story to include the enormous loss that has occurred. Through the process of consciously processing your loss and feeling the pain, you can come to a point where you can contemplate your story in a different way. You can rewrite it—yet again—with a tentative new possible ending, whether it includes having children or not. In Chapter 9, we will discuss possible paths to parenthood that you may not have considered before. We will also discuss meaningful ways to live your life even if you decide not to pursue parenthood.

EXAMPLES OF POSTTRAUMATIC GROWTH AFTER PREGNANCY LOSS

Growth can come in numerous ways. You may not even recognize how you have grown until after the fact. Growth can happen gradually and naturally as you process your loss, think about what is important to you, and set new goals.

The following are some ways that I have witnessed patients' progression after trauma. There have been times when patients don't recognize the ways in which they have grown. When I point it out to them, inevitably they smile and understand that indeed this is something to note and feel good about.

Going Public

To help others feel less isolated and ashamed about reproductive losses, many celebrities and people of renown have come forward with their own stories of loss. Meghan Markle (2020), the Duchess of Sussex, wrote an essay for the *New York Times* describing a miscarriage she experienced. She noted that although many women (and their partners) have faced the pain of pregnancy loss, the silence and shame surrounding them continues (Markle, 2020). Likewise, in her book, *Becoming*, Michelle Obama (2018) opened up about her miscarriage and feeling like a failure, and she also discussed her subsequent pregnancies using in vitro fertilization. Other celebrities have spoken out to open discussion about these losses, including Beyonce and Jay-Z, Gwyneth Paltrow, Brooke Shields, Jennifer Lawrence, Chrissy Teigen and John Legend, and the list goes on and on. Coming forward so openly about their experience has allowed others to realize they are not alone. When celebrities discuss their own pregnancy traumas, it opens doors for others to speak up as well.

More examples of people talking about their loss can be found in the U.S. Centers for Disease Control and Prevention (2021) CDC online archive and in *New York Times* (2015) reader stories. These are heartfelt accounts of people sharing narratives of having a stillbirth. Over and over, the theme of wanting to help others comes across in these stories. One woman, Kari, contributed to the stories in the CDC archive. Kari had lost her daughter, Harper, at 39.5 weeks, and she felt so much anger and guilt. She felt that she had failed to protect her baby. Because of her own experience, she wanted to do something to help other people get through the heartache.

Savannah, another patient of mine, had grown so frustrated, angry, and tired of hearing the glib and simplistic comments people made to console her after her miscarriage (things like "It was for the best," "You can have another," or "Just relax and you'll get pregnant again") that she took to social media to use her voice to educate. As Savannah stated, "I was very nervous about doing this. I wasn't sure who would read my posts and who might get offended. But I just had to do something!" She wrote about why the seemingly helpful statements were actually hurtful, and she informed people as to what would really be helpful to say:

> I let everyone know that saying "I'm so sorry for your loss" or saying something like "I can't imagine what you have gone through; I'm here for you" were the best things to communicate. And you know what? I got great feedback. Several friends posted comments thanking me and apologizing. It felt so good to put it out there.

All these examples illustrate how you can grow by sharing your experience. Taking action, such as writing about and communicating with others about your loss, can empower you. It can alter the feelings of helplessness that these kinds of losses instill and change them into strength. It can be fulfilling to know that your words can guide others through their pain and help to minimize the isolation that commonly occurs after a negative reproductive event.

Building Community

Writing about your experience is just one way to share with others. Getting involved with a support group can also lead to PTG. This was true for Maeve, who started attending an in-person peer support group for pregnancy loss. Maeve shared the following:

> The first time I went, I was really terrified. It was just weeks after our son, Peter, was born still. I really didn't know what to expect. Maybe because I was judging myself so harshly, I expected the other people there to judge me as well.

Maeve found just the opposite. The support and understanding provided by the other members of the group let her know that she was not alone.

As time went on, Maeve became more involved in the group and its organization. "I volunteered to work on the board and help set up outreach programs. This group was a life preserver for me, and I wanted to make sure other women and couples knew of its existence," she shared. Maeve's commitment to the group not only reinforced a sense of community, but it also allowed her a venue to process her grief. When new people joined, Maeve was not only able to use what she had learned to support them, but she also recognized how far she had come in her own journey of healing. "I never would have known the power of this kinship with others. It has truly changed my life," Maeve said.

Taking on New Challenges

Lucia, 34 years old, had painful periods for as far back as she could remember. She assumed it was normal, as her friends complained about their periods as well. It wasn't until she and her husband tried to have a family that she found out she had endometriosis, which explained her painful periods. *Endometriosis* is a condition where the tissue that lines the uterus also grows outside of the uterus, which can affect the ovaries and the fallopian tubes and result in fertility struggles. In Lucia's case, cysts were found on her ovaries (also known as *endometriomas*), which interfered with egg development. She was thus thrust into a medical world that she never anticipated.

> I studied history in college, and I have been teaching high school students for the past 8 years. While it has been rewarding launching these kids into the world, my husband and I were ready to have kids of our own. We just assumed it would be the next step for us. We weren't prepared to face fertility complications and so many medical interventions. The struggles to get pregnant were overwhelming.

Lucia wound up taking a leave of absence from work. She said, "It was just too difficult. I had to take so much time off for surgeries and medical issues that it just didn't make sense to keep on teaching. That was yet another blow. Everything in my life felt upended."

With more time on her hands, Lucia found herself pulled to learning more about the reproductive options open to her. "I started researching donor technology and was struck by the complex legalities involved. The issue of anonymity for the donors and the recipients was fascinating to read about, especially now when an internet search makes anonymity nearly impossible," she said. Over the course of the next year—as the reality of using an egg donor became more likely—Lucia decided to go back to school and pursue a law degree.

Returning to school, switching careers, trying a new hobby, or maybe deciding to train for and run a marathon are all examples of how people find new meaning in their life after trauma. The trauma and loss can serve as a reminder that life is short; it can also serve as a spark to tackle your proverbial bucket list. Allowing yourself to open doors that you may not have even known you were keeping closed is finding growth after your loss.

Service to Others

The theme of giving to and helping others who are dealing with reproductive loss can be seen over and over. As mentioned earlier, many people join support groups—first as a participant seeking support and then as a caregiver offering help to others. Some, as discussed, have written and shared their personal accounts so that others can learn from them. Other people have donated memory boxes to hospitals or developed fundraising campaigns to increase awareness of perinatal loss. One couple began an annual toy drive for hospitalized children. Some hospitals have created community gardens for parents to plant something in honor of their deceased child. Likewise, others sponsor a walk to remember—a ceremony for people in the community, parents, families, and friends—to come together and remember their babies who have died due to miscarriage, stillbirth, or infant death (https://nationalshare.org). These events are held all over the United States, often in October, which is National Pregnancy and Infant Loss Awareness month.

All these activities are ways of giving and receiving. In helping others, we also help ourselves. This give and take enables us to grow. Each time we do something for someone else, we also learn a little bit more about ourselves.

Self-Care and Simple Pleasures

Making big changes is not the only way to experience growth. Sometimes, simply taking note of the small, daily pleasures of life brings a sense of satisfaction. Spending time with friends and family, taking a walk in nature, and listening to music are all ways in which you can appreciate the moment. Can you challenge yourself to turn off your phone and disconnect from the blast of news and information that constantly assails us? By choosing to disengage, you can reengage with yourself. In Chapter 7, we talked about practicing *mindfulness*—that is, being present and paying attention to the moment you are in. It is a way to notice and appreciate the wonder that is in front of and all around you. This is the practice of not taking things for granted. The saying "Stop and smell the roses" is a perfect example of mindfulness. Intentionally slowing down and paying attention to what is around you is part of PTG.

Many of the examples of PTG listed earlier described ways in which people have pursued helping others. It is just as important to ensure you focus on yourself. Self-care—what is soothing and relaxing—is vital to each of us. For example, you may prefer to take a warm bath with candles lit around the tub, or perhaps curl up with a good book. Maybe getting a massage or having a spa day is what revitalizes you. What self-care looks like to you may be very different for someone else: It is the giving to yourself in a gentle and tender way that not only helps you heal from the trauma and loss but also adds to your appreciation of life. How would you soothe the baby you long to hold in your arms? Can you treat yourself with the same loving care?

Exercise 8.2 summarizes our discussion of PTG in this chapter. Consider the questions posed to discover how you may have changed, or will change, as a result of the evolution of your reproductive story.

EXERCISE 8.2. An Exercise for Your Future Self

As mentioned throughout this chapter, the concept of PTG takes time. How you feel presently may be very different from how you will feel 6 months, a year, or even 5 years from now. We've talked about how your

(*continues*)

EXERCISE 8.2. An Exercise for Your Future Self (Continued)

reproductive story has evolved over time—and what your story looks like now will be very different from what it will be like in the future. With that in mind, this exercise is really geared for your future self. Here are some questions you can ask yourself as you contemplate how you have changed, or might change, after trauma.

- Are there new things that interest me?
- How have my relationships changed?
- Do I have more compassion for others?
- Are my priorities in life different now than before the loss?
- Do I feel like I can handle stress better?
- Can I find something to appreciate every day in my life?
- How do I think about things differently?

If you can, it would be great to compare your answers today with those from your future self. What advice would you give your current self? What recommendations would you give yourself, knowing that your story is still evolving? While stories have a beginning, a middle, and an end, today you may not be able to envisage what that end may look like—including whether your story will include children or not. Whatever the future holds, you will have changed, grown, and deepened your understanding of yourself and your life with the passing of time.

SUMMARY

While at times it might seem unimaginable that anything good could come from the tragedy of your loss, it can and does. Just like in mythology where the fabled phoenix rises from the ashes of its previous life, you can emerge from your hardship with more strength, wisdom, and power than before.

No one seeks trauma in order to grow but it is undeniably true that when tragedy strikes, we evaluate ourselves and our lives in new ways. Lives can be divided into periods before and after the trauma. Research has indeed addressed these changes, citing shifts in one's self-awareness, relationships with others, and thoughts about what is meaningful in life (Tedeschi et al., 2015). Your loss may make you acutely aware of the present and not take it for granted.

In processing your loss, you reevaluate your reproductive story by asking yourself, "What do I want now, and how do I get there?" This is an opportunity to explore options in family building that you may have otherwise not thought possible. Chapter 9 ("One Story Ends, Another Begins") addresses the many new ways in which reproductive medicine has allowed people to create families, including using a donor (egg, sperm, or embryo) or surrogate, among others. It also discusses the possibility of building a family through adoption, as well as the option to remain child-free. The work involved in rewriting and editing your story is intense and comes with its own set of challenges. Growth comes from facing these challenges and taking the next steps forward.

CHAPTER 9

ONE STORY ENDS, ANOTHER BEGINS

The ideas you had about creating a family when you first started this journey are no doubt different from the reality of your current situation. Your reproductive story has taken devastating turns; as you rebuild your life, you may now be headed in directions that had been unthinkable before. This chapter will help you explore the possibilities that lie ahead—whether they include having children (or more children) or not. This is about imagining different endings to your story. Or perhaps it is better to think about contemplating new and different beginnings to the life that is unfolding in front of you.

You may not be ready to read this chapter yet. It may be too soon after your loss to contemplate another attempt at pregnancy or even consider if you want to try again. What this chapter does provide—when you are ready—is an overview of some of the possible and common medical interventions available, along with some of the legal, ethical, and financial challenges that can ensue. Although it is not possible to cover every intervention or possible option, this chapter examines procedures such as intrauterine insemination (IUI), in vitro fertilization (IVF), intracytoplasmic sperm injection (ICSI), donor technology (egg, sperm, and embryo donation), and surrogacy. We'll also focus on advances in *cryopreservation*—the freezing of eggs, sperm, and embryos—and what advances in genetic testing of embryos can tell you. Plunging into this medical world is not for everyone. In the pursuit of considering different possibilities, exploring adoption is discussed here as well. Finally, the option to remain child-free is addressed. Although this may not seem like a viable choice, hearing from people who have opted for a child-free life may allow you to see it as an opportunity for yourself.

ANALYZING THE CHOICES

When faced with life choices of such great emotional magnitude as having children, it can be helpful to create a model—a decision tree of sorts. Doing so allows you to use the analytic part of your brain by incorporating a step-by-step examination of your options and to temporarily put your feelings aside. Although this is good practice for all major decisions, it is especially helpful here because your choices now are not only about your life but also your future child's life. Knowing what is important to you, understanding what you are willing to forego, and being aware of the moral, ethical, and financial issues in the various ways of creating a family will help clarify which options will make sense for you.

Pregnancy Using Your Own Gametes

For heterosexual couples, most often the first choice is to conceive using your own gametes (i.e., your eggs or sperm and those of your partner) without having to seek medical intervention (Figure 9.1). For the LGBTQ+ community and for single parents by choice, you may want to use your own gametes, but you may also need to use a donor, a surrogate, or both to build your family (Raja et al., 2022). Regardless of your sexual orientation, if you have had a pregnancy loss, conceiving again with success is statistically high. Without factoring for age, approximately 85% of women who have had one

FIGURE 9.1. Pregnancy Using Your Own Gametes

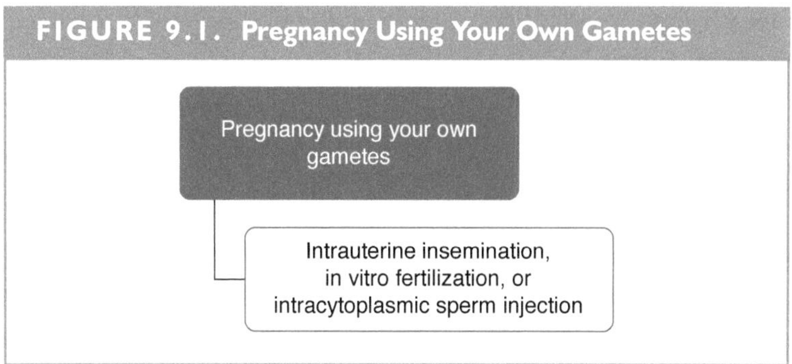

miscarriage will go on to have a healthy pregnancy (American Pregnancy Association, 2024). The statistics for women who experience a stillbirth indicate that 50% to 80% will become pregnant again (Gower et al., 2023). Conceiving again after a loss raises lots of emotions. Although you may feel joy and relief, at the same time you will likely experience dread and anxiety that you could have another loss. Chapter 7 offers strategies to help you cope with your anxiety during this time.

There are situations, though, when people need the help of medical interventions to conceive. Knowing what is available to you will help with making decisions. Next, we will review some of the common procedures. Please note that this chapter is not meant to provide medical advice; discussing these options with your doctor is essential for your care.

Intrauterine Insemination

Intrauterine insemination (also known as *artificial insemination*) is a procedure in which sperm is placed directly into the uterus using a small catheter. This procedure can improve the chances of a pregnancy by increasing the number of sperm that reach the fallopian tubes. IUI can be helpful for heterosexual couples who are struggling to conceive, using a sample of the male partner's sperm. This allows both partners to be genetically related to the resulting fetus. IUI is also used for same-sex female couples or for single women using donated sperm. It is often used as a first choice because it is less expensive and less invasive than IVF (American Society for Reproductive Medicine, 2021b).

In Vitro Fertilization

The first IVF procedure was performed in 1978, with the birth of Louise Brown in England. Since then, with refinements and advances in reproductive medicine, millions of babies have been born as a result of IVF. It is a safe and effective procedure to help couples and single women conceive. IVF is expensive. Although insurance may cover some IVF medical expenses, many policies do not cover everything, which may make it financially prohibitive for some.

Here is how IVF works: In a normal ovulatory cycle, the ovaries release follicles. One of the follicles will then develop into a fully mature egg, which has a chance of becoming fertilized and developing into a pregnancy. In an IVF procedure, a woman's ovaries are stimulated by injecting hormones (fertility drugs) to produce several mature eggs at one time, instead of just one. Through a minor surgical procedure, the eggs are then retrieved and combined with sperm in a petri dish in a laboratory to fertilize. The sperm can be from a partner—potentially creating a fully genetically related offspring—or donor sperm can be used (American Society for Reproductive Medicine, 2018).

Once a fertilized egg—or embryo—develops outside of the woman's body, it can then be tested for chromosomal anomalies. In recent years, there has been a revolution in genetic testing. Prior to 1990, testing on the fetus was done either with amniocentesis (a test that removes a sample of cells from the amniotic fluid) or chorionic villus sampling (a test that takes a sample of the placenta). These tests were conducted after a woman was pregnant.[1] Now one can test embryos in an IVF cycle, prior to transferring them into the uterus: This is known as *preimplantation genetic testing* (PGT) and is done by extracting cells from the embryo and analyzing its chromosomal makeup. It is then determined whether the biopsied cells are *euploid* (chromosomally normal) or *aneuploid* (having too few or too many chromosomes). An aneuploid embryo is less likely to lead to birth and has a greater chance of causing a miscarriage.

It would be wonderful if the results of PGT were black and white, providing people with certainty as to whether the tested embryos were healthy. Another condition, known as *mosaicism*, can lead to confusion and added stress. As an embryo develops, cells divide many times, usually with the correct number of chromosomes (23 pairs). Sometimes when they replicate, however, a mistake can happen and a cell may have one more or one less chromosome. Both normal and abnormal chromosomes can exist within the same embryo. An embryo is considered mosaic if the number of abnormal cells is between 20% and 80% (Preimplantation Genetic Diagnosis International Society, 2016). This does not mean that the embryo won't develop into a healthy baby; it depends on the specific chromosomes involved. It may be that many people living today had some mosaicism as they were developing as an embryo. We know that embryos can self-correct, discarding cells that are defective and allowing the development of a normal embryo. Consultation with a genetic counselor is necessary to help explain each unique situation.

Once an embryo has been deemed ready, it can then be transferred back into the woman's uterus. A pregnancy occurs when the

[1]Chorionic villus sampling was performed between 11 and 14 weeks of pregnancy, whereas amniocentesis was done between 15 and 18 weeks, leaving a short timeframe to consider terminating the pregnancy if genetic anomalies were found.

embryo attaches to the uterine lining and develops until birth. Although many embryos may grow in the petri dish, it is common practice to freeze them and only transfer one embryo at a time. This procedure, known as *single embryo transfer*, reduces the chance of having twins or multiple pregnancies, which can be risky for both the mother and babies, with higher chances of premature birth. Any remaining frozen embryos can be used later to add a sibling to the family if desired.

Intracytoplasmic Sperm Injection

Added to the many alphabetic abbreviations overwhelming the world of reproductive medicine is *intracytoplasmic sperm injection*, a type of IVF in which a doctor injects live sperm into eggs in a laboratory. In regular IVF, thousands of sperm are placed next to the eggs; it is left to chance whether the sperm will penetrate an egg and fertilize it. With ICSI, a single sperm is injected into the egg, thus increasing the chance of fertilization. This procedure is often used when there is male factor infertility (American Society for Reproductive Medicine, 2021a).

Benefits and Challenges of Using Intrauterine Insemination, In Vitro Fertilization, or Intracytoplasmic Sperm Injection

In the procedures just described, it is possible to create an embryo that is genetically related to partners in a heterosexual relationship. This technology allows you to experience pregnancy and childbirth, with genetically related offspring. It also allows same-sex female couples and single women, using a sperm donor, to experience pregnancy and childbirth. Although these interventions are generally considered safe and effective, they are not necessarily easy. IVF, for example, requires hormonal injections and careful monitoring for retrieval of the eggs at the optimal time. IVF may pose not only physical challenges but also psychological ones, increasing stress, anxiety, or depression. It is also expensive and not always covered partially or fully by insurance, as mentioned earlier. The cost may exclude many from even considering IVF as an option. Also, there is no guarantee that IVF will work. The success rate for IVF with tested embryos deemed suitable for transfer is approximately 50% (Society for Assisted Reproductive Technology, 2025).

The next category we'll explore is pregnancy created using either donor sperm or donor eggs. Using this technology, one can still experience pregnancy and childbirth, but not with gametes shared with your partner. Only one of you will be genetically related to the offspring.

Pregnancy With One Genetic Tie

What may have seemed like science fiction just a few decades ago is now regular practice in reproductive medicine. The use of donor eggs or donor sperm (or both) has become common, in large part because of advances in IVF and cryopreservation (the freezing of cells; Figure 9.2). If you want to have the experience of pregnancy and childbirth but cannot use your own gametes, then you might consider using a donor. Donor technology is also used to increase the odds of

FIGURE 9.2. Pregnancy With One Genetic Tie

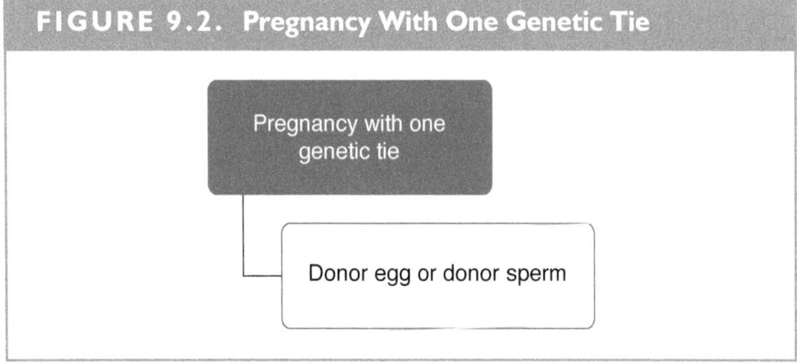

getting pregnant. For example, a 40-year-old woman using her own eggs has a 44% chance of conceiving naturally in a year, whereas a woman younger than 30 has an 85% chance to conceive. If an older woman uses eggs from a donor in her 20s, then her odds of conception are like those of the 20-something-year-old. These days, with so many women delaying childbearing, age-related fertility issues have become more common. These issues can be circumvented by using the eggs of a younger donor (Delbaere et al., 2020).

Donor insemination (DI) of sperm dates back to 1784, when Lazzaro Spallanzani performed the first successful insemination experiment using a dog (Foote, 2002). Fast-forward to the middle of the 20th century when DI began to be used in humans. A leap occurred in 1953, when the first frozen sperm was used for a human pregnancy, and thus the sperm bank industry was inaugurated (Ombelet & Van Robays, 2015). Sperm banks allow you to choose a donor based on height, hair and eye color, ethnicity, or education. You can also read a description of the donor's personality and hobbies. Now frozen sperm is regularly used by single women, lesbian couples, or heterosexual couples (either a donor's or the partner's sperm).

Compared with DI, egg or ovum donation is relatively new and more complicated. The egg donor must undergo an IVF cycle to stimulate her ovaries and then retrieve the viable eggs. Those eggs are then fertilized in a petri dish with the partner's or donor's sperm. As with traditional IVF, the resulting embryos may be tested and then transferred back into the woman's body.

For members of the LGBTQ+ community or single parents by choice, finding and using a donor is often the first step to starting a family. For most heterosexual couples, using donor technology, whether egg or sperm, is usually not their first choice; rather, they consider it after they have dealt with reproductive trauma once or multiple times. The use of a donor can be intertwined with feelings of grief. Couples are faced with letting go of their reproductive stories of how they expected to conceive, and they need to create a new story that incorporates a third party (the donor) into their ideas of conception.

Numerous questions and concerns can be raised by using donor technology. How do you choose a donor? What characteristics of the donor should you consider? These questions are often followed by a slew of others: Who is the "real" parent? If you are not biologically related to the child, will you be able to form an attachment with and love that child? Do you tell your child of their origins? If so, how and when? Will they feel different from other children? How will your family react? What if this goes against your religious or cultural traditions? The following examples try to answer some of these questions.

How Do You Choose a Donor?

Darcy, 38, was recovering from her third pregnancy loss in 2 years. She and her husband, Ken, 39, were naturally devastated and had to consider what to do next. Darcy shared the following:

> I can't keep doing this. I am drained to the point that it is impacting everything. When I first wake up in the morning, I feel okay, but then within seconds, the dark clouds start to roll in and my mood sinks.

At Darcy's last doctor's appointment, her obstetrician raised the idea of using an egg donor. "Ken and I have been mulling this over, knowing that our odds for getting pregnant and having it stick will go up dramatically. But . . .," she said, falling silent. It was clear she was weighing their options but was not yet ready to make a decision.

"What are some of your worries?" I gently asked.

"I had a hard enough time picking my husband," Darcy joked. "And now I'm supposed to find someone he can have a child with?"

She grew serious. "Does he want someone who looks like me? Or will this fulfill some fantasy of his?"

"Choosing a donor can feel very much like a dating match website, and that can feel bizarre. And kind of arbitrary," I agreed. I then emphasized the following point:

> But Ken will be having a child with *you*. It is *you* that he wants to raise a child and build a family with. Finding someone who resembles you in some respects—your looks, your education, your interests—that is often how people choose.

Another worry people may have is that the donor (whether it is an egg or sperm donor) will have some parental rights. Rest assured, this is not the case. Donors are considered biological contributors, not parents. Although some parents and their donor may choose to have an ongoing relationship, the donor has no legal or financial obligations in raising the child.

Will I Feel Like a Parent?

Darcy was also worried about whether she would be considered a real parent. She shared the following:

> I guess I'm also worried about how people will react. I mean, are they going to think of Ken as the "real" parent and me as—I don't know what—an understudy or a substitute teacher? Am I a placeholder until the authentic parent shows up? Will this child even love me? Or will I love them?

In trying to reassure Darcy that she would be just as real a parent as Ken, I pointed to the literature in the field of epigenetics. *Epigenetics* is the study of how environmental factors can influence cells without changing the DNA sequence. The science informs us that the woman who carries the pregnancy has a direct influence on what genes are turned on and off, affecting the fetus's development (Zuccarello et al., 2022). The actual sequence of DNA does not change, but environmental factors, such as the mother's diet, hormones, and microbes that live inside or on the body (e.g., bacteria, fungi, or viruses), all affect the developing fetus. Although she may not use her own gametes, the woman carrying the pregnancy still has a biological connection with the developing fetus.

It was also helpful for Darcy to understand what adoptive parents experience. The literature on adoption talks about the idea of *parental claiming*, the process of feeling that you can parent—in fact, you have the right to parent—a child who is not genetically your own. I also told Darcy about research conducted with egg donor mothers who go through the same process (Imrie et al., 2020). At first, they may feel that this baby is not really theirs to parent; through nurturing care, they feel this baby is completely a member of the family.

"You are not alone in having these worries," I assured Darcy. "It's all about attachment. Did you know that many people who have biological children don't necessarily feel that attachment immediately?" I asked her. I then shared the following details about attachment:

> It's really not all about genetics. Attachment happens when your baby cries and you feed them and then, magically, they are content. It happens again when they are upset, and you change their diaper. It happens yet again when they need to be held, and you do, and it soothes them. This process also comforts you—you are able to take care of their needs. And it happens countless times in one day—over and over your caring for them makes them feel good and then you feel good. You and your baby build this bond that no one else has. That's what attachment really is.

Who Does the Baby Look Like?

Feelings of being an imposter parent can be exacerbated when people talk about who your baby looks like. Before a baby's personality emerges, people commonly comment on not only how adorable the baby is but also who the baby looks like. Geri and Craig used donor sperm and gave birth to Michael, who was 5 months old. Even though they chose a sperm donor with Craig's hair color and eye color; it appeared, at least for now, that Michael's features were more like Geri's.

"It is driving me crazy," Geri began. "Why do people think it is funny to wonder if I hooked up with a delivery driver?" She turned to Craig and asked, "How do those jokes make you feel?"

"Well," Craig began, "I know it's said in jest, but it does sting a bit." He continued, "I try to joke back, saying that he looks like me when he's sleeping—like an angel. I mean, lots of kids look more like one parent than the other, so why do they need to dwell on this?"

We discussed the concept known as *resemblance talk*, which are the comments people make about a child's physical resemblance to their parents or other family members. When looks are discussed, the implication is that the child is genetically related, making legitimate the child's place in the family. For donor-conceived children (whether by sperm or egg donation) and their parents, resemblance talk can feel threatening. Parents worry that their child may feel stigmatized and as if they are somehow different. There is the fear that their child won't feel a part of the family unit. Parents also worry about their own legitimacy as parents, as previously discussed with the notion of parental claiming. Creating a family in this way raises many issues that just don't exist for traditional family configurations.

How Do We Talk to Our Child About Their Birth Story?

One of the biggest concerns parents of donor-conceived children have is whether to disclose the story of their birth and, if so, when and how.

Geri and Craig were torn about this. When Geri and Craig were counseled prior to using the donor, they were advised to disclose to their child or children the truth about their conception—and they agreed. However, that was before they had Michael, this real little person who woke up smiling 9 times out of 10 and could be cajoled into giggles even when he was grumpy. Now they weren't sure what to do.

"I mean," Geri began, "Michael had no choice in this. We have burdened him with being different right from the start. I just want things to be normal for him."

Craig agreed. Michael was asleep on his lap, snuggled in his arms. "Sometimes I wonder if we did the right thing. He's going to be encumbered by our decision for his whole life. If he doesn't know about the donor, he'll be able to be just like everyone else," Craig said as he held Michael closer. I continued,

> As I listen to both of you, it's clear that you want the best for Michael. Your love for him is palpable. I know that whatever you decide to do will be in his best interest. I do think it's important, though, to explore the downsides to not having this conversation with him. Tell me who else knows that you used a donor to have him.

That grabbed their attention. Wide-eyed, they went down the list of individuals who knew about their reproductive journey: their parents, Craig's brother, and Geri's two best friends. "We asked them not to tell anyone else . . . but I know my mother told her sister," Geri added sheepishly. "I mean, it's not a secret, but we don't need the whole world to know." I raised the following point of view they likely had not considered:

> Of course not, but you don't want Michael to find out about his beginnings from someone other than you two. And you need to take into consideration the proliferation of genetic testing these

> days and revelations about one's DNA. What if he were to find out that way? It's a matter of truth-telling and trust—essential for a solid family foundation. You also need to consider who Michael might be romantically involved with in the future. I know it's far off at this point, but you don't want him to accidentally get involved with a half-sibling. Also, there might be issues that come up with the donor's health. These might directly affect Michael, and he should be able to have that knowledge.

Geri and Craig looked at each other with trepidation. The silence was broken when Craig said, "Okay, I get it. But how do we do it, and when? He certainly won't understand what we're talking about now." They both looked down at Michael with concern. I explained,

> Some people wait until they think their child is old enough to understand. The problem with that is it often gets put off indefinitely. Other families talk about it even before their child is verbal. Kind of like planting a seed to be discussed again and again. It's kind of "always knowing" his birth story. No doubt he'll have questions as he gets older: This is not a one-time conversation. But starting it now allows you to feel more at ease with it. And then if issues do come up for him, you'll be there to help him. That's what all parents should do—whether they've used a donor or not.

Michael stirred a bit as Craig passed him into Geri's arms. "Alright, kiddo," she began. "Listen up! Your dad and I had some help in creating you. And we are so happy we did!"

Pregnancy With No Genetic Ties

There are more possibilities to be had in this brave new world of reproductive medicine. Here we'll discuss two other options: embryo donation and embryo creation (Figure 9.3). Both allow a woman to carry the pregnancy and give birth to her child but without her or her partner's genetic material.

Embryo Donation

When people go through an IVF cycle, excess embryos can result, leaving people in a conundrum of what to do with them. At the beginning of an IVF cycle, the hope is for as many viable embryos as possible. Once family building is complete, however, there still may be leftover frozen embryos, and the decision of how to handle them can raise financial, ethical, and legal questions. The embryos can remain frozen, but there are fees to do so and space is limited; they really shouldn't be left on ice forever.

One option is to donate excess embryos for scientific research. They can also be thawed and discarded. If people think of their embryos as children or potential children, they may struggle with donating them to science or allowing for their destruction. Indeed, the notion that frozen embryos should be entitled to the same rights as someone who is born complicates legal implications for reproductive medicine. As of this writing, the issue of personhood is being

FIGURE 9.3. Pregnancy With No Genetic Ties

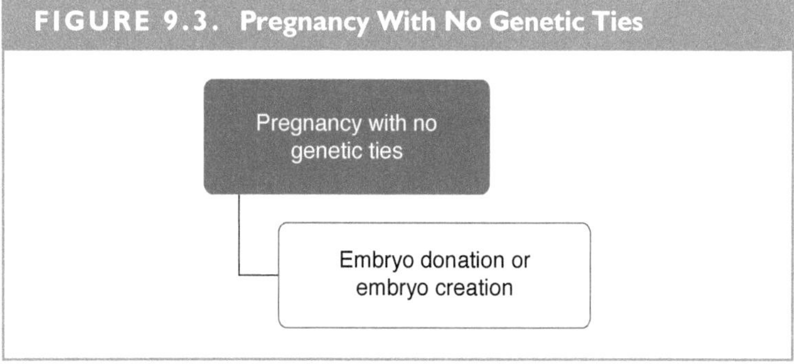

debated in the courts and legislative bodies in the United States (Letterie & Fox, 2023). One ramification for providers could be that they may legally be forced to perform embryo transfers that have a low probability of leading to a live birth. Patients would then be faced with the anguish of loss (American Society for Reproductive Medicine, 2025).

Yet another option for frozen embryos is to donate them to an infertile couple or individual to create a family. This approach allows the recipient woman the opportunity to experience pregnancy and childbirth but with no genetic ties (except as discussed earlier, with the ability to affect how genes are turned on and off). When a child is born through embryo donation, they will likely have a full biological sibling being raised in another family. All the issues that families go through with donor-conceived children apply here as well, including worries about resemblance talk, parental claiming, and disclosure (not only to the child but also to other people). Indeed, the American Society for Reproductive Medicine (2023c) recommended that both sets of families undergo psychological evaluations and receive psychological support to ensure the welfare of the child or children, especially if the families are known to each other. The American Society for Reproductive Medicine also recommended seeking legal counsel, especially because laws on this topic vary from state to state. Legal agreements between the embryo donors and the embryo recipients need to be executed to make clear who the parents are. The families, tied together forever through their children, can establish if and how they manage contact with each other in the future.

Embryo Creation

It is also possible to create embryos using donor eggs and donor sperm. In this case, the egg donor goes through an IVF process; the eggs are then fertilized in a petri dish with donor sperm. The resulting embryo or embryos can then be transferred into a woman, who will carry and give birth to her child. Unheard of just a few years ago, there are now donor embryo banks that create embryos and match them with recipients. The donors in these programs are anonymous; the embryos are formed by using donor eggs and donor sperm to try to match the characteristics of the recipients. Would-be parents get to know about the donor's medical history, ethnic and family background, and a bit about the donor's personality. In many cases, if multiple embryos are created, they can be shared with other families, thus producing full genetic siblings who will be raised in separate families.

The issue of disclosure to these children is important, as it is with any use of donor eggs or donor sperm. In all cases, it is the welfare of the child or children that is of utmost concern, especially as it relates to *consanguinity* (i.e., two closely related individuals mating with each other or, in other words, having an unintentional incestual relationship). It is possible for half-siblings who were created with the same donor to meet and have a child of their own. For example, a sperm donor could create many half-siblings, raised in different families, without the half-siblings knowing that the others existed. Although other countries limit the number of children a sperm donor can create, the United States does not have any laws regulating this. The Donor Sibling Registry (DSR), available online (https://donorsiblingregistry.com), was developed to address the burgeoning population of donor-conceived children and to enable them to contact others who share their genetic ties. Through the DSR program, people can register with their donor number and are contacted if someone else posts with the same donor number. Not only can people connect with each other, but they can also share and update medical information with each other. The mission of the DSR is the belief that everyone has the right to know about their biological origins.

Surrogacy

Surrogacy is the process of a woman bearing a child to give to another woman or couple to raise (Figure 9.4). It has been around since biblical times, most notably in the Book of Genesis, where we understand that Sarah and her husband, Abraham, struggled with infertility (*King James Bible*, 1769/2025, Genesis 11:30, 15:2–4). As the story goes, Sarah wanted her servant, Hagar, to have a child with Abraham, which Hagar would then give to Sarah (*King James Bible*, 1769/2025, Genesis 16:1–16). Abraham impregnated Hagar, and a son, Ishmael, was born. The subsequent relationship between Sarah and Hagar was fraught with hostility and jealousy. This type of surrogacy—when a woman carries a child using her own gametes on behalf of another person or couple—is known as *traditional surrogacy* (TS). In essence, in this type of surrogacy arrangement, the surrogate is both the egg donor and the biological mother. Because of the bond between biological mother and child as well as the potential difficulty in relinquishing the child, this type of surrogacy arrangement is not advised. In fact, in most U.S. states, traditional surrogates have legal rights to the child; in many states, TS is illegal. For the legal and emotional reasons stated, the American Society for Reproductive Medicine does not recommend TS (Kim, 2020).

FIGURE 9.4. Parenthood With Possible Genetic Ties

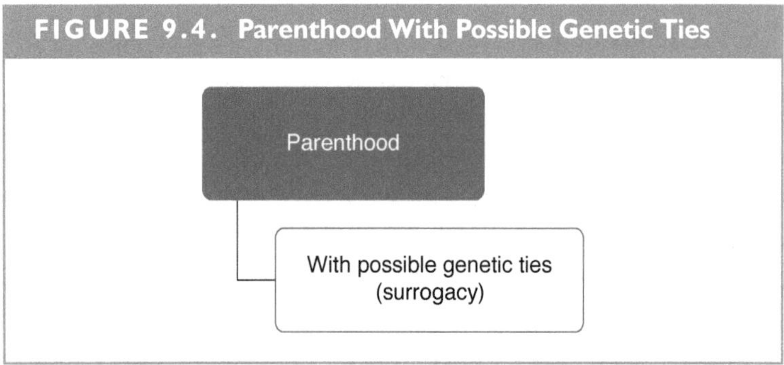

Since the development of IVF, TS is less preferred compared with another form of surrogacy referred to as a *gestational carrier arrangement*. Here, the *gestational carrier* (or surrogate) has no genetic ties to the baby. She does not provide the egg but carries the pregnancy to term and gives birth, making the legal process much less complicated. The individual or couple who will then raise the child and are legally recognized as the parents are called *intended parents*, a term commonly used in the realm of surrogacy. Intended parents may be a single man or a same-sex male couple who want to have children. Likewise, an intended parent may be a woman who has struggled with infertility or is unable to carry a child, including a single woman or a woman in a same-sex female couple or a heterosexual couple.

In many cases in which an individual or couple uses a gestational carrier, at least one intended parent provides genetic material. That is, an individual or couple may use their own egg or a donor egg and their own sperm or donor sperm in an IVF cycle, and the resulting embryo is then transferred into the surrogate. In some cases, if a woman is unable to carry a pregnancy but can produce eggs and her partner can produce sperm, then genetic material from both intended parents can be used. Some people use a gestational carrier if an intended parent cannot carry a pregnancy because of uterine problems or if she has had a hysterectomy or other health issues. A gestational carrier is also used by gay men who would like to create a family. Although the financial arrangements may be prohibitive—with costs including surrogate compensation, legal fees, and medical expenses—this is an opportunity for the intended parents to have a baby that would otherwise be impossible.

For the surrogate, giving of herself, her body, and her time can feel amazingly rewarding. In the most selfless way possible, she is helping another couple or individual who would otherwise not be able to experience parenthood to fulfill their dream of having a child. Surrogates often feel an enormous sense of pride in their role. One gestational carrier said, "I am changing the world by doing this!" The relationship that forms between the gestational carrier and the intended parents will differ from one arrangement to another, but the potential for connection and appreciation of each other in this process is vast. For both the intended parents and the gestational carrier, the anxiety surrounding this enormous decision can feel overwhelming. Here's a snippet of some feelings shared in therapy sessions that describe the emotions of both parties:

Gestational Carrier: Wow! I was just matched with a couple! This is real! We are planning to meet next week. I loved being pregnant, but I really don't know what this is going to feel like. Signing up for this feels so exciting and a little bit crazy!

Intended Parent: OMG! We were matched with a surrogate, and we'll meet her next week! We hope she won't mind us coming to appointments with her, and we hope she'll take good care of herself and our baby. It's so intense to trust a complete stranger with carrying our child. We are so excited, but it feels a little crazy!

As you can see, there is excitement and trepidation among all parties involved. This is a long journey, one in which there may be bumps along the way. Both the gestational carrier and the intended parents may have expectations that may not be met. For example, sometimes intended parents want constant updates about the pregnancy, want to know about the gestational carrier's activities, and may even want to know what she is eating. Intended parents may also worry if the gestational carrier is traveling. These situations may cause the gestational carrier to feel as if she is not being trusted to take care of herself. Another misunderstanding may occur regarding doctor's appointments and medical tests. The gestational carrier may have to partake in drug screening and more medical testing before and throughout the pregnancy than she did in her own biological pregnancy. In a case I saw in my practice, a surrogate fell during the pregnancy. Although she claimed she was fine, the intended parents insisted that she get checked out by her doctor. Tensions grew when the gestational carrier refused to seek medical attention, again insisting that there was nothing wrong. While it is impossible to predict every misunderstanding or conflict that might occur, keeping the dialogue and conversation open among all parties involved can help smooth over any misunderstandings. Having regular check-ins can make this a fulfilling experience unlike any other.

Adoption

As long as humans have been in existence, so too has adoption (Figure 9.5). It is a way for biological parents who cannot care for their child to relinquish them to the care of another family. Most often, birth parents decide on adoption as a result of financial constraints, knowing that they cannot adequately care for the child. It

FIGURE 9.5. Parenthood With No Genetic Ties

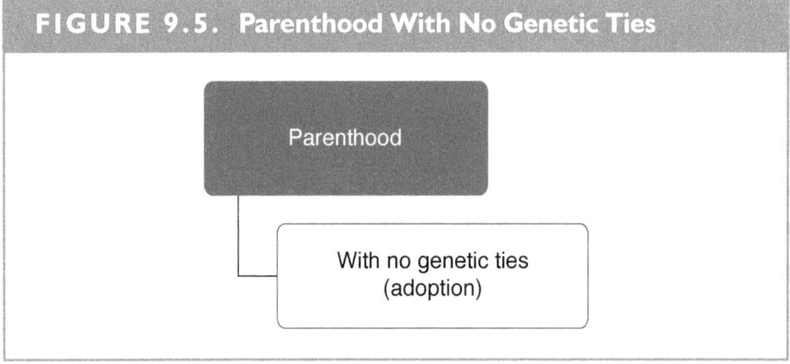

is estimated that 40% of birth mothers already have other children and choose to relinquish a child not only for the sake of that child but also for the family they already have (Smith, 2006). It is an emotionally complex decision that needs to be grieved just as any pregnancy loss is. The decision often falls solely on birth mothers. They wonder if they are doing the right thing, feeling a sense of loss and isolation. Will their baby be safe and well cared for? Will they be able to keep in touch and have contact with their child as they grow up? What will the child think of them? Although birth mothers may bear the brunt of the decision, research suggests that birth fathers also wonder about the child and may have persistent feelings of shame and inadequacy (Clapton, 2019).

On the other side, parents who choose to adopt also face many emotional considerations. Many adoptive parents may have tried to conceive on their own, they may have faced infertility or pregnancy loss (or both), or they may not want to venture into the medical world of assisted reproduction or may not have had success if they have. Although some people choose to adopt altruistically, others may see adoption as a last resort or as a backup plan if everything else has failed (Daniluk & Hurtig-Mitchell, 2003). Adoptive parents may wonder if they will be able to bond with their child. They may worry that the child will not think of them as their real parents. However, as discussed previously, attachment is not necessarily about genetics or biology; rather, it comes from the daily caring for a child, meeting their needs, and providing love and nurturance to them.

There are so many questions to consider regarding adoption. Do you adopt domestically or internationally? Do you go through an agency or adopt privately? Are you willing to adopt an older child or a child of a different ethnicity than your own? What does an open adoption really look like? It is beyond the scope of this book to delve into all the complexities of adoption. Talking to other parents who have adopted can provide an enormous amount of information and may quell some of the normal anxiety that arises. What is most important to remember is that at the end of this process, you will get to be a parent.

When you think about it, both birth parents and adoptive parents have had to radically rethink their reproductive stories. For everyone involved, there is a lot to contemplate, and having counseling and guidance throughout the process is important. The bottom line that needs to be considered is, as always: What is in the best interest of the child? The adopted child may have interest in and curiosity about their birth story and their birth parents, or they may not. It is also possible that feelings will change over time. Adoption is a lifelong process for everyone involved—the birth parents, the adoptive parents, and the child or children.

Remaining Child-Free

The difference between being child-free by choice and child-free not by choice is huge, even though the resulting circumstance (i.e., a life without raising children) is the same. Although it may not seem obvious, those who are child-free by choice have a reproductive story that examines and questions what life would be like with or without children. Their decision may be influenced by their own personal beliefs, social and economic factors, or environmental considerations, such as the worry about bringing children into the world under treacherous conditions (climate change, political unrest, economic instability, etc.). A child-free life has been considered aberrant behavior in the past. It is frequently associated with being nonconformist and selfish. Both men and women may be criticized for being self-centered as well as being unfeminine or unmanly. This trend is changing, however, with a growing number of people choosing to be child-free.

Because you are involuntarily childless, you have come to this place in your life through much heartache. This is clearly not the way you envisioned your life would be or how your reproductive story would unfold. To feel criticized in any way for being child-free only adds to the pain. It may be helpful for you to have ready answers available in your emotional toolbox in case you are asked about your parental status. It can ease the discomfort to be prepared if a person you are meeting for the first time asks, "Do you have any kids?" While this is a common conversation starter, it may land with a twinge—or more—of emotional pain.

If the societal message is that parenthood is equated with fulfillment in life, does that mean that living a child-free life is devoid of purpose or joy? The answer is a resounding no. Even if childlessness was not your choice, opportunities and relationships that might otherwise not have been possible can be pursued. You can change the narrative on this, opening doors—both big and small—that you may not have thought possible before. As discussed in Chapter 8, one of the measures of posttraumatic growth is new possibilities. There are so many ways to feel fulfilled in life. For example, maybe you pursue a passion that positively impacts the next generation. One child-free man became a docent at a local science and natural history museum, delighted by being able to explain exhibits to visiting children. A woman who was an avid reader opted to volunteer in her community, reading to children and getting them excited by literature. If you have nieces, nephews, or godchildren, you might spend more time with them, give them more attention, and perhaps spoil them in ways their parents cannot. This is another way of providing nurturance to the children in your life.

Perhaps you engage more deeply in the work that you already do, which is another way to feel fulfillment. On the other hand, without the demands of raising a family, maybe you want to switch careers, go back to school, or pursue a business idea that you've been thinking about. It is not possible here to list the many avenues that might be open to you, but the realization that you can seek out other possibilities for yourself and make a difference can bring much satisfaction and joy. Another positive change that couples describe is a deepening connection in their relationship. One man commented, "Now that we are not spending all our energy—and money—on trying to create a family, we have more time and resources to do the things we enjoy."

Turning the narrative from a loss to a win will not occur overnight. You are grieving not only the baby or dream that you have lost but also the life you had expected. No doubt there will be moments where sadness and grief feel overwhelming. Acknowledging these feelings, and sitting with them, is really okay. The goal is not to push them aside, but to rewrite your reproductive story with a different ending and acknowledge that your worth is about how you engage with the life you have.

WHAT IS RIGHT FOR US?

If you are feeling overwhelmed by the multitude of possibilities available to you and all the implications involved—whether it is finding alternative ways to become parents or deciding to remain child-free—you are not alone. How do you make these kinds of decisions? How do you envision your life moving forward? One woman, Didi, said,

> I can't imagine what it will be like if we stop trying. I've defined myself and my life over the past 3 years trying to have a baby. After months of disappointment when I didn't get pregnant and had two miscarriages in the middle of all that, I have been consumed.

Didi wasn't ready to call it quits, but she wasn't sure how to proceed.

If you find yourself in this position—not knowing if, when, or how to move forward—it can help to imagine yourself in the future. What might it feel like a year from now? Five years? Ten years? Can you imagine different endings to your reproductive story? What would it feel like to parent a child who was not genetically related to you, to your partner (if you have one), or to both of you? How might you handle a situation where you feel questioned about your status as a parent? What if you are comfortable accepting one avenue to pursue, but your partner is not? If you feel as if your partner is blocking you—in a sense, being a gatekeeper—resentments and frustrations will no doubt flare up. Now more than ever you need to understand your own feelings as well as each other's feelings. Sometimes it can help to start with what you do agree on—for example, that you want to have a family—and then work backward from there. What are the most acceptable ways of pursuing this dream together? What are the things that frighten you and your partner? What you don't want is for one of you to just give in to the other's wishes. That may only engender anger and bitterness as you move forward in your lives.

This may be a time when you decide to seek therapy. Talking with friends and family can be helpful, but they may chime in with their own opinions, causing more confusion. This is why talking with a neutral third party who does not have a stake in a specific outcome can be most effective. Having a safe space to air your feelings, and likewise allowing your partner to air theirs, is part of the healing. Being able to listen to your partner's story and reflect on your own will allow both of you to weigh the plusses and minuses of each possibility.

SUMMARY

Your loss has taken its toll. No doubt you feel worn down by this struggle. This may be a challenging time for you and your relationship, but it can also be an exciting time as you contemplate a way forward—whether it includes children or not. Your reproductive story has not gone as you had anticipated, and the path forward may feel strange and rocky. One thing to remember is that there is no one right answer: There is no one-size-fits-all solution to your ongoing reproductive story.

This chapter has suggested some possible ways of editing your story, rewriting it such that you can find a path forward. You may feel pressed to find a solution immediately, but it takes time to consider these choices. Because your case is unique to you (and your partner, if you have one), it is imperative that you discuss all these possibilities and hopes with your medical provider.

EPILOGUE

THE END OF THE STORY

Simply put, the arc of any story has a beginning, a middle, and an end. As a story begins, we meet various characters, see how they develop and transform over time, and finally come to a resolution at the finale. Fairy tales, for example, often start with "Once upon a time," followed by struggles with witches, evil spells, or difficult heroic tasks, and conclude with "happily ever after."

Your reproductive story—as discussed throughout this book—follows a similar pattern in many ways. We know how it started. We can look back at our own childhood and understand how the idea of becoming a parent is woven throughout our lives. It is so deeply ingrained that we may take it for granted; it is just something that "is." The story grows and develops as we do—from childhood, to adolescence, and into adulthood. The backdrop to this story usually includes the notion that you can have children if you want them and build a family of your own.

This book finds you in the middle of your reproductive story. It goes without saying that the struggles you have experienced—the trauma and losses that have occurred—are not what you expected. Your hopes and dreams of having a baby have been shattered. Feelings about yourself and your relationships have also taken a beating, perhaps adding doubts about your worthiness and increasing a sense of insecurity. This moment—this middle part of your story—may feel like it will never end. You are likely feeling stuck in limbo as you grieve, questioning the very meaning of life. "Why has this happened to me?" you may cry. "How can I move on?"

One way to understand the possibilities that lie ahead is to think about different endings to your reproductive story. Imagine, if you can, different possible avenues that your reproductive story could take. Would you consider using a donor, for example, or would you want to pursue adoption? Thinking about how each of these potential strategies might feel allows you to see what might work for you. What frightens you? What feels overwhelming? How do financial considerations come into play? Does your cultural or religious background play a part in how you feel? Making sense of our thoughts and feelings is how we all reach decisions and make choices throughout life. The point here is that you are in control of this part of the story. You (and your partner) get to decide what to pursue—what avenues you may take to create a family—or not.

When you are stuck in the middle, you may not be able to imagine that your life will continue and change. You may not be able to predict the end of the story, but you will not be trapped in this place forever—the story will come to an end whether you decide to have children (or more children) or not. That doesn't mean that you won't feel sad or upset; the grief that comes with pregnancy losses is lifelong. The intensity of all your bad feelings will fade, but you have been forever changed by this heartbreaking experience.

As with all stories, this book has now come to an end. My hope is that it has provided you with insight and has helped you through a very difficult part of your life. As discussed, people grow out of adversity. How this trauma and loss has changed you may be yet to unfold, but your focus on yourself and those around you will no doubt lead to growth. You will get through this.

I leave you with the words often attributed to the great Joseph Campbell:[1]

> We must be willing to let go of the life we have planned so as to accept the life that is waiting for us.

[1]Joseph Campbell (1904–1987) was a writer, teacher, and scholar specializing in exploring the human condition through mythology and comparative religion.

RESOURCES

The following is a list of some resources that you may find helpful through your journey of healing from pregnancy loss.

American Society for Reproductive Medicine (https://www.asrm.org) is dedicated to the advancement of reproductive medicine. The organization's website includes a section for reproductive patients, which offers fact sheets and informational booklets on a wide array of subjects. You can also find a listing of mental health providers here.

Compassionate Friends (https://www.compassionatefriends.org) provides support to bereaved families after the death of a child.

Donor Sibling Registry (https://donorsiblingregistry.com) helps donor-conceived people connect with their half-siblings and learn about their genetic origins.

International Stillbirth Alliance (https://www.stillbirthalliance.org) aims to raise awareness globally to prevent stillbirth and newborn death.

Mommies Enduring Neonatal Death (M.E.N.D.) (https://www.mend.org) offers in-person and virtual support groups for both men and women.

***New York Times* "Stillbirth: Your Stories"** (https://www.nytimes.com/interactive/2015/health/stillbirth-reader-stories.html) features accounts written by parents who have navigated stillbirth and want to share their insights.

Postpartum Support International (PSI) (https://postpartum.net) provides mental health support for pregnancy, postpartum, and after loss. Support is also available for postadoption depression and anxiety.

Rachel's Gift (https://www.rachelsgift.org) offers free virtual support groups for families coping with miscarriage, stillbirth, and infant death.

RESOLVE (https://resolve.org) was established in 1974 and is dedicated to support and advocacy for those who are faced with challenges in building a family. It is a resource for support groups (in person or virtual).

Return to Zero H.O.P.E. (https://rtzhope.org) provides support and resources for anyone who has experienced infertility, miscarriage, stillbirth, or infant death. This organization also offers support to those who have had to terminate a desired pregnancy, or have had a failed surrogacy or a failed adoption.

Share Pregnancy and Infant Loss Support (https://nationalshare.org) provides support groups, both in person and online. This organization also offers memorial events, such as the Share Walk for Remembrance and Hope.

U.S. Centers for Disease Control and Prevention CDC Family Stories Archive (https://archive.cdc.gov/#/details?url=https://www.cdc.gov/ncbddd/stillbirth/family-stories/index.html) features stories written by and for those who have experienced a stillbirth.

Walk With Me (https://www.walkwithme-nonprofit.org) is devoted to giving practical, financial, and emotional support to those who have experienced the death of their child either prior to birth or shortly after.

REFERENCES

Alvarez-Calle, M., & Chaves, C. (2023). Posttraumatic growth after perinatal loss: A systematic review. *Midwifery*, *121*, 103651. https://doi.org/10.1016/j.midw.2023.103651

American College of Obstetricians and Gynecologists. (2022). *FAQs: Exercise during pregnancy*. https://www.acog.org/womens-health/faqs/exercise-during-pregnancy

American College of Obstetricians and Gynecologists Committee on Obstetric Practice. (2020). Physical activity and exercise during pregnancy and the postpartum period: ACOG Committee Opinion, Number 804. *Obstetrics and Gynecology*, *135*(4), e178–e188. https://doi.org/10.1097/AOG.0000000000003772

American Pregnancy Association. (2024). *Pregnancy after miscarriage*. https://americanpregnancy.org/getting-pregnant/pregnancy-loss/pregnancy-after-miscarriage/

American Psychiatric Association. (2022). *Diagnostic and statistical manual of mental disorders* (5th ed., text rev.). https://doi.org/10.1176/appi.books.9780890425787

American Society for Reproductive Medicine. (2012). *Age and fertility: A guide for patients*. https://www.reproductivefacts.org/news-and-publications/fact-sheets-and-infographics/age-and-fertility-booklet/

American Society for Reproductive Medicine. (2018). *Assisted reproductive technologies: A guide for patients*. https://www.reproductivefacts.org/news-and-publications/fact-sheets-and-infographics/assisted-reproductive-technologies-booklet

American Society for Reproductive Medicine. (2021a). *Intracytoplasmic sperm injection (ICSI): Fact sheet.* https://www.reproductivefacts.org/news-and-publications/fact-sheets-and-infographics/intracytoplasmic-sperm-injection-icsi/

American Society for Reproductive Medicine. (2021b). *Intrauterine insemination (IUI): Fact sheet.* https://www.reproductivefacts.org/news-and-publications/fact-sheets-and-infographics/intrauterine-insemination-iui/

American Society for Reproductive Medicine. (2023a). *Reproductive facts: Defining infertility.* https://www.reproductivefacts.org/news-and-publications/fact-sheets-and-infographics/defining-infertility/

American Society for Reproductive Medicine. (2023b). *Reproductive facts: Ectopic pregnancy.* https://www.reproductivefacts.org/globalassets/_rf/news-and-publications/bookletsfact-sheets/english-pdf/ectopic_pregnancy_factsheet.pdf

American Society for Reproductive Medicine. (2023c). *Reproductive facts: Embryo donation: What should I know?* https://www.reproductivefacts.org/globalassets/_rf/news-and-publications/bookletsfact-sheets/english-pdf/embryo_donation_what_should_i_know_factsheet.pdf

American Society for Reproductive Medicine. (2025). *ASRM position statement on personhood measures.* https://www.asrm.org/advocacy-and-policy/fact-sheets-and-one-pagers/asrm-position-statement-on-personhood-measures

Angarita, A. M., Johnson, C. A., Fader, A. N., & Christianson, M. S. (2016). Fertility preservation: A key survivorship issue for young women with cancer. *Frontiers in Oncology*, *6*(6), 102. https://doi.org/10.3389/fonc.2016.00102

Ayalti, E. D. E., & Bayraktar, S. (2017). Examination of factors related with posttraumatic growth in infertile individuals. *International Journal of Social Science and Education Research*, *3*(4), 1216–1232.

Bailey, S., Bailey, C., Boivin, J., Cheong, Y., Reading, I., & Macklon, N. (2015). A feasibility study for a randomised controlled trial of the Positive Reappraisal Coping Intervention, a novel supportive technique for recurrent miscarriage. *BMJ Open*, *5*(4), e007322. https://doi.org/10.1136/bmjopen-2014-007322

Baker, J. E. (2001). Mourning and the transformation of object relationships. *Psychoanalytic Psychology*, *18*(1), 55–73. https://doi.org/10.1037/0736-9735.18.1.55

Berghella, V., & Saccone, G. (2017). Exercise in pregnancy! *American Journal of Obstetrics and Gynecology*, *216*(4), 335–337. https://doi.org/10.1016/j.ajog.2017.01.023

Bhat, A., & Byatt, N. (2016). Infertility and perinatal loss: When the bough breaks. *Current Psychiatry Reports*, *18*(3), 31. https://doi.org/10.1007/s11920-016-0663-8

Blos, P. (1967). The second individuation process of adolescence. *Psychoanalytic Study of the Child*, *22*(1), 162–186. https://doi.org/10.1080/00797308.1967.11822595

Brendel, A. M., & Kennedy, R. (2023, January 20). *Implications of abortion laws for fertility services*. Goodwin Procter LLP. https://www.goodwinlaw.com/en/insights/publications/2023/01/01_20-implications-of-abortion-laws-for-fertility-services

Brownlee, K., & Oikonen, J. (2004). Toward a theoretical framework for perinatal bereavement. *British Journal of Social Work*, *34*(4), 517–529. https://doi.org/10.1093/bjsw/bch063

Cann, A., Calhoun, L. G., Tedeschi, R. G., Kilmer, R. P., Gil-Rivas, V., Vishnevsky, T., & Danhauer, S. C. (2010). The Core Beliefs Inventory: A brief measure of disruption in the assumptive world. *Anxiety, Stress, and Coping*, *23*(1), 19–34. https://doi.org/10.1080/10615800802573013

Clapton, G. (2019). Against all odds? Birth fathers and enduring thoughts of the child lost to adoption. *Genealogy*, *3*(2), 13. https://doi.org/10.3390/genealogy3020013

Colarusso, C. A. (1990). The third individuation: The effect of biological parenthood on separation-individuation processes in adulthood. *Psychoanalytic Study of the Child*, *45*(1), 179–194. https://doi.org/10.1080/00797308.1990.11823516

Cuenca, D. (2023). Pregnancy loss: Consequences for mental health. *Frontiers in Global Women's Health*, *3*, 1032212. https://doi.org/10.3389/fgwh.2022.1032212

Daniluk, J. C., & Hurtig-Mitchell, J. (2003). Themes of hope and healing: Infertile couples' experience of adoption. *Journal of Counseling and Development*, *81*(4), 389–399. https://doi.org/10.1002/j.1556-6678.2003.tb00265.x

Delbaere, I., Verbiest, S., & Tydén, T. (2020). Knowledge about the impact of age on fertility: A brief review. *Upsala Journal of Medical Sciences*, *125*(2), 167–174. https://doi.org/10.1080/03009734.2019.1707913

Dobbs v. Jackson Women's Health Organization, 597 U.S. ___ (2022). https://www.oyez.org/cases/2021/19-1392

Doka, K. J. (1989). Disenfranchised grief. In K. J. Doka (Ed.), *Disenfranchised grief: Recognizing hidden sorrow* (pp. 3–11). Lexington Books/ Free Press.

Doka, K. J., & Martin, T. L. (2011). Grieving styles: Gender and grief. *Grief Matters*, *14*(2), 42–45.

Eldeib, D. (2023, March 23). *Federal study calls U.S. stillbirth rate 'unacceptably high' and recommends action*. ProPublica. https://www.propublica.org/article/stillbirths-rate-nih-cdc-prevention-research

Food and Drug Administration v. Alliance for Hippocratic Medicine, 602 U.S. ___ (2024). https://www.oyez.org/cases/2023/23-235

Foote, R. H. (2002). The history of artificial insemination: Selected notes and notable. *Journal of Animal Science*, *80*(Suppl. 2), 1–10.

Freud, S. (2000). Recommendations to physicians practicing psychoanalysis. In J. Strachey (Ed. & Trans.), *The standard edition of the psychological works of Sigmund Freud* (pp. 1–120). Hogarth Press. (Original work published 1912)

Galst, J. P. (2018). The elusive connection between stress and infertility: A research review with clinical implications. *Journal of Psychotherapy Integration*, *28*(1), 1–13. https://doi.org/10.1037/int0000081

Genovese, H. G., & McQueen, D. B. (2023). The prevalence of sporadic and recurrent pregnancy loss. *Fertility and Sterility*, *120*(5), 934–936. https://doi.org/10.1016/j.fertnstert.2023.08.954

Ghasemi, M., Kordi, M., Asgharipour, N., Esmaeili, H., & Amirian, M. (2017). The effect of a positive reappraisal coping intervention and problem-solving skills training on coping strategies during waiting period of IUI treatment: An RCT. *International Journal of Reproductive Biomedicine*, *15*(11), 687–696.

Gold, K. J., Leon, I., Boggs, M. E., & Sen, A. (2016). Depression and posttraumatic stress symptoms after perinatal loss in a population-based sample. *Journal of Women's Health*, *25*(3), 263–269. https://doi.org/10.1089/jwh.2015.5284

Goldbach, K. R., Dunn, D. S., Toedter, L. J., & Lasker, J. N. (1991). The effects of gestational age and gender on grief after pregnancy loss. *American Journal of Orthopsychiatry*, *61*(3), 461–467. https://doi.org/10.1037/h0079261

Gosso, Y., & Carvalho, A. M. A. (2013, June). Play and cultural context. In R. E. Tremblay, M. Boivin, R. De V. Peters, & P. K. Smith (Eds.), *Encyclopedia on early childhood development*. https://www.child-encyclopedia.com/play/according-experts/play-and-cultural-context

Gower, S., Luddington, J., Khosa, D., Thaivalappil, A., & Papadopoulos, A. (2023). Subsequent pregnancy after stillbirth: A qualitative narrative analysis of Canadian families' experiences. *BMC Pregnancy and Childbirth*, *23*(1), 208. https://doi.org/10.1186/s12884-023-05533-5

Greenfeld, D. A., Diamond, M. P., & DeCherney, A. H. (1988). Grief reactions following in-vitro fertilization treatment. *Journal of Psychosomatic Obstetrics and Gynaecology*, *8*(3), 169–174. https://doi.org/10.3109/01674828809016784

Grocher, K., & Gerrits, T. (2023). A racially and culturally sensitive approach to fertility counseling. In S. N. Covington (Ed.), *Fertility counseling: Clinical guide* (2nd ed., pp. 183–194). Cambridge University Press.

Hendrix, T., Roncoroni, J., Magdamo, B., Whitaker, S., Zareba, K., & Grieco, N. (2023). Stigma, social support, and decision satisfaction in terminations of pregnancy for medical reasons. *Women's Health Reports*, *4*(1), 271–279. https://doi.org/10.1089/whr.2022.0092

Hughes, P., Turton, P., Hopper, E., & Evans, C. D. H. (2002). Assessment of guidelines for good practice in psychosocial care of mothers after stillbirth: A cohort study. *The Lancet*, *360*(9327), 114–118. https://doi.org/10.1016/S0140-6736(02)09410-2

Hurd, W. W. (2016). Waiting to conceive after an early pregnancy loss. *Obstetrics and Gynecology*, *127*(2), 197–198. https://doi.org/10.1097/AOG.0000000000001276

Hydén, L.-C. (2010). Identity, self, narrative. In M. Hyvärinen, L. C. Hydén, M. Saarenheimo, & M. Tamboukou (Eds.), *Studies in narrative: Vol. 11. Beyond narrative coherence* (pp. 33–47). John Benjamins Publishing Company. https://doi.org/10.1075/sin.11

Imrie, S., & Golombok, S. (2018). Long-term outcomes of children conceived through egg donation and their parents: A review of the literature. *Fertility and Sterility*, *110*(7), 1187–1193. https://doi.org/10.1016/j.fertnstert.2018.08.040

Imrie, S., Jadva, V., & Golombok, S. (2020). "Making the child mine": Mothers' thoughts and feelings about the mother–infant relationship in egg donation families. *Journal of Family Psychology*, *34*(4), 469–479. https://doi.org/10.1037/fam0000619

Jaffe, J. (2024). *Reproductive trauma: Psychotherapy with clients experiencing infertility and pregnancy loss* (2nd ed.). American Psychological Association. https://doi.org/10.1037/0000400-000

Jaffe, J., & Diamond, M. O. (2011). *Reproductive trauma: Psychotherapy with infertility and pregnancy loss clients*. American Psychological Association. https://doi.org/10.1037/12347-000

Kabat-Zinn, J. (2021). The liberative potential of mindfulness. *Mindfulness*, *12*(6), 1555–1563. https://doi.org/10.1007/s12671-021-01608-6

Khoury, B., Sharma, M., Rush, S. E., & Fournier, C. (2015). Mindfulness-based stress reduction for healthy individuals: A meta-analysis. *Journal of Psychosomatic Research*, *78*(6), 519–528. https://doi.org/10.1016/j.jpsychores.2015.03.009

Kim, H. H. (2020). Selecting the optimal gestational carrier: Medical, reproductive, and ethical considerations. *Fertility and Sterility*, *113*(5), 892–896. https://doi.org/10.1016/j.fertnstert.2020.03.024

King James Bible. (2025). *King James Bible Online: Book of Genesis*. https://www.kingjamesbibleonline.org/Genesis (Original work published 1769)

Kingdon, C., Givens, J. L., O'Donnell, E., & Turner, M. (2015). Seeing and holding baby: Systematic review of clinical management and parental outcomes after stillbirth. *Birth*, *42*(3), 206–218. https://doi.org/10.1111/birt.12176

Krawczyk, A., Kretek, A., Pluta, D., Kowalczyk, K., Czech, I., Radosz, P., & Madej, P. (2022). Gluten-free diet: Remedy for infertility or dangerous trend? *Ginekologia Polska*, *93*(5), 422–426. https://doi.org/10.5603/GP.a2021.0223

Krosch, D. J., & Shakespeare-Finch, J. (2017). Grief, traumatic stress, and posttraumatic growth in women who have experienced pregnancy loss. *Psychological Trauma: Theory, Research, Practice, and Policy*, *9*(4), 425–433. https://doi.org/10.1037/tra0000183

Kübler-Ross, E. (1969). *On death and dying*. Macmillan.

Leon, I. G. (1996). Revising psychoanalytic understandings of perinatal loss. *Psychoanalytic Psychology*, *13*(2), 161–176. https://doi.org/10.1037/h0079646

Letterie, G., & Fox, D. (2023). Legal personhood and frozen embryos: Implications for fertility patients and providers in post-*Roe* America. *Journal of Law and the Biosciences*, *10*(1), lsad006. https://doi.org/10.1093/jlb/lsad006

Lindemann, E. (1944). Symptomatology and management of acute grief. *The American Journal of Psychiatry*, *101*(2), 141–148. https://doi.org/10.1176/ajp.101.2.141

Lovell, A. (2001). The changing identities of miscarriage and stillbirth: Influences on practice and ritual. *Bereavement Care*, *20*(3), 37–40. https://doi.org/10.1080/02682620108657527

MacNaughton, H., Nothnagle, M., & Early, J. (2021). Mifepristone and misoprostol for early pregnancy loss and medication abortion. *American Family Physician*, *103*(8), 473–480.

Mahler, M., Pine, F., & Bergman, A. (1975). *The psychological birth of the human infant*. Basic Books.

Markle, M. (2020). The losses we share. *New York Times*. https://www.nytimes.com/2020/11/25/opinion/meghan-markle-miscarriage.html

Matthews, T. J., & Ventura, S. J. (1997). Birth and fertility rates by educational attainment: United States, 1994. *Monthly Vital Statistics Report*, *45*(10 Suppl.), 1–20.

McCreight, B. S. (2004). A grief ignored: Narratives of pregnancy loss from a male perspective. *Sociology of Health & Illness*, *26*(3), 326–350. https://doi.org/10.1111/j.1467-9566.2004.00393.x

Miller, S., Wherry, L. R., & Foster, D. G. (2020). What happens after an abortion denial? A review of results from the Turnaway Study. *AEA Papers and Proceedings*, *110*, 226–230. https://doi.org/10.1257/pandp.20201107

Nam, S. K., Chu, H. J., Lee, M. K., Lee, J. H., Kim, N., & Lee, S. M. (2010). A meta-analysis of gender differences in attitudes toward seeking professional psychological help. *Journal of American College Health*, *59*(2), 110–116. https://doi.org/10.1080/07448481.2010.483714

Nandi, P., Roncari, D. M., Werner, E. F., Gilbert, A. L., & Ramos, S. Z. (2024). Navigating miscarriage management post-*Dobbs*: Health risks and ethical dilemmas. *Women's Health Issues*, *34*(5), 449–454. https://doi.org/10.1016/j.whi.2024.05.004

National Academies of Sciences, Engineering, and Medicine Committee on Reproductive Health Services. (2018). *The safety and quality of abortion care in the United States*. National Academies Press. https://www.ncbi.nlm.nih.gov/books/NBK507237/

New York Times. (2015, June 26). *Stillbirth: Your stories*. https://www.nytimes.com/interactive/2015/health/stillbirth-reader-stories.html

Nietzsche, F. (2008). *Twilight of the idols.* (D. Large, Trans.). Oxford University Press. (Original work published 1888).

Norcross, J. C., & Phillips, C. M. (2020). Psychologist self-care during the pandemic: Now more than ever. *Journal of Health Service Psychology*, *46*(2), 59–63. https://doi.org/10.1007/s42843-020-00010-5

Obama, M. (2018). *Becoming*. Crown.

Ombelet, W., & Van Robays, J. (2015). Artificial insemination history: Hurdles and milestones. *Facts, Views & Vision in Obstetrics & Gynecology*, 7(2), 137–143.

Pasch, L. A., Holley, S. R., Bleil, M. E., Shehab, D., Katz, P. P., & Adler, N. E. (2016). Addressing the needs of fertility treatment patients and their partners: Are they informed of and do they receive mental health services? *Fertility and Sterility*, *106*(1), 209–215.e2. https://doi.org/10.1016/j.fertnstert.2016.03.006

Paul, M. S., Berger, R., Berlow, N., Rovner-Ferguson, H., Figlerski, L., Gardner, S., & Malave, A. F. (2010). Posttraumatic growth and social support in individuals with infertility. *Human Reproduction*, *25*(1), 133–141. https://doi.org/10.1093/humrep/dep367

Practice Committee of the American Society for Reproductive Medicine. (2019). Fertility preservation in patients undergoing gonadotoxic therapy or gonadectomy: A committee opinion. *Fertility and Sterility*, *112*(6), 1022–1033. https://doi.org/10.1016/j.fertnstert.2019.09.013

Practice Committee of the American Society for Reproductive Medicine. (2023). *Definition of infertility: A committee opinion.* https://www.asrm.org/practice-guidance/practice-committee-documents/definition-of-infertility/

Preimplantation Genetic Diagnosis International Society. (2016, July 10). PGDIS position statement on chromosome mosaicism and preimplantation aneuploidy testing at the blastocyst stage. *PGDIS Newsletter.* https://www.pgdis.org/docs/newsletter_071816.html

Raja, N. S., Russell, C. B., & Moravek, M. B. (2022). Assisted reproductive technology: Considerations for the nonheterosexual population and single parents. *Fertility and Sterility*, *118*(1), 47–53. https://doi.org/10.1016/j.fertnstert.2022.04.012

Ramos, C., & Leal, I. (2013). Posttraumatic growth in the aftermath of trauma: A literature review about related factors and application contexts. *Psychology, Community & Health*, 2(1), 43–54. https://doi.org/10.5964/pch.v2i1.39

Rando, T. A. (1985). Bereaved parents: Particular difficulties, unique factors, and treatment issues. *Social Work, 30*(1), 19–23. https://doi.org/10.1093/sw/30.1.19

Rando, T. A. (1986). *Parental loss of a child.* Research Press.

Ranji, U., Diep, K., Gomez, I., Sobel, L., & Salganicoff, A. (2024, July 29). Health policy issues in women's health. In Altman, D. (Ed.), *Health policy 101.* KFF. https://www.kff.org/health-policy-101-health-policy-issues-in-womens-health/?entry=table-of-contents-introduction

Rocca, C. H., Samari, G., Foster, D. G., Gould, H., & Kimport, K. (2020). Emotions and decision rightness over five years following an abortion: An examination of decision difficulty and abortion stigma. *Social Science & Medicine, 248*, 112704. https://doi.org/10.1016/j.socscimed.2019.112704

Rooney, K. L., & Domar, A. D. (2018). The relationship between stress and infertility. *Dialogues in Clinical Neuroscience, 20*(1), 41–47. https://doi.org/10.31887/DCNS.2018.20.1/klrooney

Ryninks, K., Wilkinson-Tough, M., Stacey, S., & Horsch, A. (2022). Comparing posttraumatic growth in mothers after stillbirth or early miscarriage. *PLoS One, 17*(8), e0271314. https://doi.org/10.1371/journal.pone.0271314

Schwartz, S. E. O., Benoit, L., Clayton, S., Parnes, M. F., Swenson, L., & Lowe, S. R. (2022). Climate change anxiety and mental health: Environmental activism as buffer. *Current Psychology, 42*, 1–14. https://doi.org/10.1007/s12144-022-02735-6

Schwerdtfeger, K. L., & Shreffler, K. M. (2009). Trauma of pregnancy loss and infertility for mothers and involuntarily childless women in the contemporary United States. *Journal of Loss and Trauma, 14*(3), 211–227. https://doi.org/10.1080/15325020802537468

Sherman, D. W., Alfano, A. R., Alfonso, F., Duque, C. R., Eiroa, D., Marrero, Y., Munecas, T., Radcliffe-Henry, E., Rodriguez, A., & Sommer, C. L. (2024). A systematic review of the relationship between social isolation and physical health in adults. *Healthcare, 12*(11), 1135. https://doi.org/10.3390/healthcare12111135

Smith, P. J., & Merwin, R. M. (2021). The role of exercise in management of mental health disorders: An integrative review. *Annual Review of Medicine, 72*(1), 45–62. https://doi.org/10.1146/annurev-med-060619-022943

Smith, S. L. (2006). *Safeguarding the rights and well-being of birthparents in the adoption process*. Evan B. Donaldson Adoption Institute.

Society for Assisted Reproductive Technology. (2025). *All SART member clinics—2023 retrieval and transfer tables*. https://www.sartcorsonline.com/EmbryoOutcome/PublicSARTOutcomeTables?reportingYear=2023&ClinicPKID=0

Stroebe, M., Finkenauer, C., Wijngaards-de Meij, L., Schut, H., van den Bout, J., & Stroebe, W. (2013). Partner-oriented self-regulation among bereaved parents: The costs of holding in grief for the partner's sake. *Psychological Science*, *24*(4), 395–402. https://doi.org/10.1177/0956797612457383

Stroebe, M., & Schut, H. (1999). The dual process model of coping with bereavement: Rationale and description. *Death Studies*, *23*(3), 197–224. https://doi.org/10.1080/074811899201046

Tedeschi, R. G., & Calhoun, L. G. (2004). Posttraumatic growth: Conceptual foundations and empirical evidence. *Psychological Inquiry*, *15*(1), 1–18. https://doi.org/10.1207/s15327965pli1501_01

Tedeschi, R. G., Calhoun, L. G., & Groleau, J. M. (2015). Clinical applications of posttraumatic growth. In S. Joseph (Ed.), *Positive psychology in practice: Promoting human flourishing in work, health, education, and everyday life* (2nd ed., pp. 503–518). John Wiley & Sons.

Triplett, K. N., Tedeschi, R. G., Cann, A., Calhoun, L. G., & Reeve, C. L. (2012). Posttraumatic growth, meaning in life, and life satisfaction in response to trauma. *Psychological Trauma: Theory, Research, Practice, and Policy*, *4*(4), 400–410. https://doi.org/10.1037/a0024204

U.S. Centers for Disease Control and Prevention. (2021, October 4). *CDC archive: Family stories*. https://archive.cdc.gov/#/details?url=https://www.cdc.gov/ncbddd/stillbirth/family-stories/index.html

U.S. Centers for Disease Control and Prevention. (2025, May 9). *Data and statistics on stillbirth*. https://www.cdc.gov/stillbirth/data-research/index.html

U.S. Department of Labor. (n.d.). *Family and Medical Leave Act*. https://www.dol.gov/agencies/whd/fmla

Waugh, A., Kiemle, G., & Slade, P. (2018). What aspects of post-traumatic growth are experienced by bereaved parents? A systematic review. *European Journal of Psychotraumatology*, *9*(1), 1506230. https://doi.org/10.1080/20008198.2018.1506230

Winograd, M. (2017). *Understandings the predictors of posttraumatic growth among those with a history of a reproductive trauma* (Publication No. 2319) [Doctoral dissertation, Seton Hall University]. Seton Hall University Dissertations and Theses.

Wise, E. H., Hersh, M. A., & Gibson, C. M. (2012). Ethics, self-care and well-being for psychologists: Reenvisioning the stress-distress continuum. *Professional Psychology, Research and Practice*, *43*(5), 487–494. https://doi.org/10.1037/a0029446

Yu, Y., Peng, L., Chen, L., Long, L., He, W., Li, M., & Wang, T. (2014). Resilience and social support promote posttraumatic growth of women with infertility: The mediating role of positive coping. *Psychiatry Research*, *215*(2), 401–405. https://doi.org/10.1016/j.psychres.2013.10.032

Zhang, X., Deng, X., Mo, Y., Li, Y., Song, X., & Li, H. (2021). Relationship between infertility-related stress and resilience with posttraumatic growth in infertile couples: Gender differences and dyadic interaction. *Human Reproduction*, *36*(7), 1862–1870. https://doi.org/10.1093/humrep/deab096

Zuccarello, D., Sorrentino, U., Brasson, V., Marin, L., Piccolo, C., Capalbo, A., Adrisani, A., & Cassina, M. (2022). Epigenetics of pregnancy: Looking beyond the DNA code. *Journal of Assisted Reproduction and Genetics*, *39*(4), 801–816. https://doi.org/10.1007/s10815-022-02451-x

INDEX

ABOUT THE AUTHOR

Janet Jaffe, PhD, clinical psychologist, has devoted her career to helping others navigate the pitfalls and anguish that can occur on the road to parenthood. She works with patients in private practice, has trained countless mental health professionals in the United States and internationally, and has written and lectured extensively on the topic, both for professionals and patients. She is informed not only by years of academic scholarship but also from her personal experience. She knows from the inside what it means to want to build a family, and what happens when those hoped-for dreams come crashing down—whether due to miscarriage, stillbirth, infertility, or other neonatal trauma. She also knows what it takes to move forward and rebuild from these unimaginable losses. Titles by Janet Jaffe include *Unsung Lullabies: Understanding and Coping With Infertility* (with Drs. Martha and David Diamond), *Reproductive Trauma: Psychotherapy With Infertility and Pregnancy Loss Clients* (with Dr. Martha Diamond), and *Reproductive Trauma: Psychotherapy With Clients Experiencing Infertility and Pregnancy Loss*.